Born to Be Beautiful

Donna Kennedy

Contents

Acknowledgments

I want to thank: my mother and father, Maureen and Padraig Kennedy, for being my pillars of strength throughout my life; my soulmate, Pat Slattery, who gave me the gift of our beautiful baby boy, and who brings a smile to my face every day; Ashton, for lighting up my life in every way; Chris, Keith and Jason Slattery for being loving brothers; Joan Slattery for being such a lovely grandmother; my family and Pat's family, for being so loving; Raymund King and Daniela Cuellar for their invaluable advice and kindness; and Isabel Rodriguez Valerón and Idaira Villalba Reyes, for being so supportive to my baby's development.

I also want to thank the professionals who took such good care of me throughout my pregnancy at Limerick Maternity Hospital, particularly: Professor Cotter, Suzie Coombs, Helen Madigan, Laura Whelan, Joanne Moylan, Joanne Teehan, Joanna Desmond, Angela O'Farrell, Mary, Murphy, Linda Molloy, Mary McCoy, Fionnuala Ryan, Maria Gibbons, Maeve Mortell, Carmel Higgins and Angela Culligan.

Finally, I want to make sure to thank: Dr Deirdre

Collins, for being there throughout my life; Caroline McDonagh, Isabel Corral, Audrey McMahon, Lorraine McMorrow, Raphael and Pat Mullally, John Flynn and Ger Sheahan for all their support and kindness; Sabine La Fotógrafa Pelirroja and Chris Ernst for the cover photo and design; Una Williams for photography; all the people who have attended my seminars and completed my workshops; and Seán O'Keeffe and his fantastic team at Liberties Press.

Introduction

How is it that books on pregnancy always focus on the baby, not the mother, when common sense might tell us that the mother's well-being and happiness are fundamental to her baby's well-being and happiness? It's as if, when the pregnancy is confirmed, mommy fades away. That is not okay. In fact, if you ask me it's just plain crazy.

Think about it. You are the lifeline to your baby. Without you, there is nothing. It is essential, therefore, that you love and care for yourself – during and after pregnancy! Through the course of this book, you will learn to do just that! In fact, you will learn how you can look and feel amazing every day of your life. Remember this, happy mommy, happy baby.

'Having a baby is one of the most exciting, magical things that will ever happen to you.' If only I had a cent for every time I was told that when I became pregnant! But it's true: having a baby is one of the best things you will ever experience. I cannot even come close to describing how it felt to experience my baby kicking for the first time or to see him gazing up at me when he was born. It was beyond incredible.

Now, had that been the only thing people said to me when I became pregnant I would have been quite happy. But it seems that when an opportunity arises, some people aren't able to resist the temptation to tell you all the horror stories, especially their own. If your pregnancy is anything like mine, you will be led to believe that pregnancy, although a beautiful experience, will result in you losing your identity, having less self-confidence and becoming overweight. No sooner had my pregnancy been confirmed than the comments started coming: 'You can say goodbye to life as you know it.' 'Having a baby takes away your independence.' 'You can forget wearing those jeans again.' 'Enjoy that flat tummy while it lasts!'

I must be honest with you: although I was so happy to be pregnant and to know my baby was getting bigger and stronger inside me, constantly hearing such things from women who had already become mothers made me nervous about what could very easily be the new me. After all, they had been through the experience, so who was I to contradict them? Maybe I was just supposed to accept that I would end up as the woman they were describing.

I had visions of feeling trapped and upset at having to put my life on hold, disappointed that I couldn't do the things I loved anymore. I saw myself getting loads of stretch marks and ballooning like the blueberry girl, Violet Beauregarde, from *Willy Wonka and the*

Chocolate Factory, skin stretching to the point of explosion, and then struggling to get my figure back after I had my baby. I could see myself going from a confident woman to a self-doubting one.

I didn't like it one bit. I liked my life, I liked my independence, I liked my jeans and I liked my tummy. I didn't want a transformation! However, I didn't want to look overambitious at the end of my pregnancy either, deluded into thinking I could be anything but what they were describing, especially since they were all saying pretty much the same thing.

Many women believe they will inevitably have to experience certain things as a result of having a baby, and so they just accept it. They accept that they will no longer feel confident about themselves or their bodies, and they accept that pregnancy will leave them physically scarred for life. Isn't it lucky for you and me that I don't believe our destiny is set in stone!

You see, my pregnancy was planned months before I became pregnant, so I had the opportunity to research pregnancy and mommy issues in advance of giving birth. I was determined to defy my apparent fate and look and feel exactly as I wanted to post pregnancy, regardless of what other women were saying. Of course, not yet a mom, I had limited knowledge of the actual pregnancy experience but, at the time, I did have a very good understanding of nutrition and biology, so I had something solid to start with. I researched the ins and outs of pregnancy and what to expect during and after it. I figured if I knew what might happen I could steer in the direction of what I wanted to happen, obviously staying healthy in the process. I looked in depth at what women across the globe were experiencing and doing, everything from the stuff most of us already know, to old secret traditions handed down through generations. I even researched chemistry.

Using my knowledge and research, I decided to create a practical pregnancy plan so that my baby and I would really enjoy the pregnancy experience and would come out the other side of it looking and feeling amazing. Of course, as life would have it, it was not to be done without difficulty. Looking back now, I can nearly hear the laughter of life in the wind: 'Let's give Donna a real challenge. We'll make her baby BIG! A big, stripy belly guaranteed.' And so I gave birth to a 9.2-pound (4.23-kilogramme) baby boy. But I haven't a single stretch mark, I am in shape and I feel amazing. What's more, my baby is strong, healthy and has a smile that would light up a Christmas tree.

So, with my little bundle of joy by my side, I can say with certainty that it's a total myth that you have to look or feel anything less than amazing post pregnancy. It is also a myth that your life changes for the worse. It can be even more amazing than it was before pregnancy. I am living proof of it. And trust me, there's nothing special about me that would allow nature to spare me. If anything, I was given some extra challenges.

First, I have epilepsy so my pregnancy wasn't a straightforward experience. Second, post-pregnancy weight gain and stretch marks are common in my family.

So how did I maintain my self-confidence during and after pregnancy? How did I ensure a good figure? Well, I didn't attend any support groups, and I didn't starve or diet. I didn't work the treadmill, I didn't have any genetic alterations and my baby isn't a contortionist. I simply have information most women don't, and I used that information during and after pregnancy. I will share it all with you in this book – everything from how I looked after my emotional well-being to how I prevented stretch marks and got the body I wanted.

You see, when we become pregnant, and especially after we give birth, it's all too easy to let things slip. It's easy to forget that we are amazing, to forget sometimes that we even matter. It's like we go into full-blown mommy mode, focusing solely on baby, and leave our sense of self behind. After all, we have our babies to consider, right? Well, here's the thing: children learn by example and if you teach your child from day one that looking after yourself and feeling amazing is a good thing, they are likely to do the same.

1
You Matter

When I was pregnant, I saw so many mothers (both pregnant mothers and those who had already given birth) struggle with the idea of taking care of themselves, almost as though it was self-indulgent and uncaring. How could a mother possibly focus on herself and love her baby at the same time? We need to put things into perspective and get real. Taking care of *yourself* is essential to the health and happiness of your baby. Your baby *needs* a happy, healthy mom, and the only way you can be that happy, healthy mom is if you take care of yourself. When you're on a flight, what do the air hosts say you need to do if there's a sudden loss of cabin pressure? Please attend to your own mask first. And why do they say that? When you look after yourself, you are in a better position to look after others, that's why. Being your best is one of the kindest things you can do for yourself, your baby and everyone around you. Your baby wants you to look and feel amazing. The very notion of compromising your own needs and 'letting yourself go' because you are a mom is ridiculous. The truth is, not taking care of yourself is uncaring.

Our babies come into this world knowing this to be true. Getting our needs met as a human being is a necessity if we are to grow and be at our best, physically or emotionally. When our babies are born, they innately know to cry to tell us what they need, and when they get it they smile up at us with doting eyes and gooh-gah smiles to make sure we don't forget to meet their needs the next time. Do you think that happens by accident? We were designed to live fully and be the best we can be. We were designed to get our needs met. Even something as basic as a plant knows that getting its needs met is essential! If you don't give it water it strips the soil of all moisture. If you deprive it of sunlight it twists itself towards any glimmer of light it can find. A plant will only bloom if it gets what it needs; ignore it and it will look like a dried-up, miserable weed. And surely we are more intelligent than plants? The simple fact is taking care of ourselves and being the best we can be is what we were born to do. It is not something to feel bad about or ignore.

My wish for you is that you look and feel absolutely amazing now and always and to be the best you can be in every way. I want you to wake up in the morning with a smile, glad to be alive and happy in the knowledge that you are a worthwhile person who deserves everything amazing that life has to offer, during pregnancy and after it. I want you to be able to look in the mirror, feel 'wow' and celebrate who looks back at you, inside and out. And you are totally capable of making this happen. Think about it: you had the ability to create a baby! Life coming from another life, there is nothing more powerful or impressive. Can you imagine the results you will get when you really put your conscious mind to implementing the *Born to Be Beautiful* pregnancy plan?

Identifying Your Starting Point

If you are to get where you want to be you must have a starting point. Like going on a journey, if you want to get to a destination it's useful to know where you are now, where you want to be and what the best route is to get there. It makes things straightforward. I will help you identify exactly what you want your outcome to be, and I will show you the best route to get there, but first we must identify your starting point, no matter how undesirable you think it is.

Some women define their starting point as 'a disaster', 'disappointing', 'less than average', 'hopeless', 'fat', 'self-conscious', etc., whether they are pregnant or have already given birth. Everyone has their own way of describing their situation. I don't know how you would describe your current situation but whatever it may be, just acknowledge it for what it is and don't beat yourself up about it. We will be going well beyond criticising ourselves and we will be stepping into a productive way of thinking and behaving so that you will get results. But our first step must be to assess where we're at right now.

The Wheel of Human Needs

So that we do not waste any time, I would like you to do the following exercise now. This exercise is purely to ascertain your starting point; it is not an exercise of criticism of any kind. Its purpose is purely to acknowledge what is currently happening in your life and that is all. To get your results you must do three things:

1. You must understand your needs as they exist.

2. You must rate where you are now.

3. You must make take the steps that I outline in this book (having consulted with your doctor where applicable).

At this stage, I want you to simply read the list of needs that I have outlined here and ask yourself how each need applies to you and your life right now. Ask yourself whether each need is being met in balance (the goal is to create a sense of equilibrium in each area of our lives so that there is calm and not chaos), and then, later, we will rate each one on a scale from one to ten. Please note that most people do not have all their needs met in balance (many don't even know what their needs are) so don't freak out if, when you identify and rate your needs, things look hopeless. I don't know anyone who scores a ten on everything – many don't score a ten on anything – but rating your situation in this way will help you get results and get them fast.

Physical Needs

Our physical needs are perhaps the most obvious to us. They are the basis of human survival and it's important they are met in balance.

- **Shelter**: Having a roof over our heads is something every human being deserves and needs. It doesn't need to be fancy but we do need it and so do our babies. In the event you don't have a roof over your head, it is vital that you seek assistance as soon as possible.

- **Fresh air**: Our brains require a constant flow of oxygen to function normally. If our brain or our baby's brain does not get enough oxygen then it can cause serious impairments in cognitive skills, as well as in physical, psychological and other functions. Therefore, it is essential, especially during and post pregnancy, that we expose ourselves to lots of fresh air every day. Walking is a good way to do so.

- **Good nutrition**: This is essential to a healthy pregnancy and an amazing you! Eat well, have proper, full meals, and always work with your body, not against it. We will discuss this in depth later on, in the *Born to Be Beautiful* food plan.

- **Clean water**: Next to oxygen, clean water is the most essential element to human life; the body usually cannot survive longer than a few days without it (a maximum of a week). Water is essential to the functioning of every single cell and every organ system in your body (and in your baby's body). It makes up more than two-thirds of the weight of the human body: the brain is seventy-five percent water, blood is eighty-three percent water, bones are twenty-two percent water, muscles are seventy-five percent water and lungs are ninety percent water. Water is needed for the efficient elimination of waste products through the kidneys, regulation of body temperature (through perspiration), cushioning of the joints, good digestion and metabolism and delivery of nutrients and oxygen to all cells in the body. It facilitates all of the chemical processes which occur in the body. A decrease of as little as two percent in our body's water supply can have harmful effects and cause symptoms of dehydration, such as daytime fatigue, excess thirst, fuzzy memory, difficulty focusing on tasks, light-headedness and nausea. So drink up!

- **Sleep**: When we have babies, our sleep patterns certainly change. A full night's sleep just isn't always possible or practical, especially if you are breastfeeding. However, we are not robots; we need sleep to function properly. If we do not get enough sleep it can affect our mental and physical health, which is bad for us and bad for our babies. For this reason, it is very important that you sleep as often as you can. As a rule of thumb, for the first few months, you should take a couple of naps during the day when your baby is napping. Ideally, you would get support in looking after your baby, such as sharing night feeds or making room in the day to allow you to get sleep, but if this doesn't happen you need to make sleep a priority any time you can get it.

- **Movement**: Regular physical activity is one of the most important things we can do for our health and physical appearance. Later, you will learn the *Born to Be Beautiful* movement plan, which you can easily incorporate into your day. It will have you looking amazing in a very short period of time.

Emotional Needs

Most people do not take care of their emotional needs or even know what they are. However, ignoring or compromising our emotional needs is what causes most of our problems. Let's look at what's important.

- **Safety and security**: In general, we feel safe when we feel competent to deal with what is happening in our lives, and we feel secure when we know that our environment (emotional, financial, etc.) is stable. Needless to say, pregnancy can throw all this up in the air, leaving us in fear of the unknown. It is very common to feel nervous about both pregnancy and motherhood, so if you feel nervous it is perfectly normal and understandable. After all, there is no rule book for it – and for good reason, in my opinion, as no two children are the same. Simply love and care for your baby and trust your intuition. If they smile often for the right reasons, you are doing a good job! Your health care provider will advise you on the specifics so you feel secure in the knowledge that everything is okay. You'll be shown how and when to feed your baby, etc. and regular health checks will be made available to you. Be sure to ask questions – even the ones you are embarrassed about – and to seek assistance if you need it.

- **Control and autonomy**: Every human being needs to have a sense of order and control, whether in deciding what to eat for dinner or in planning for the future. However, during and after pregnancy, life can feel a bit out-of-control, especially if we fear the unknown or don't like change, which is the case for the majority of the population. It's important, therefore, to create a plan for when the baby arrives, so that you can enjoy being a mother. This is different for everyone but as a general guideline, you could have your basic items bought before the baby arrives, such as the contents of a baby bag, baby clothes and bibs, a stroller, etc. You don't need to go out and get everything, the basics are fine. You could also plan feeds in advance and, once the baby is born, write down key phone numbers in case you need them (doctor, health nurse, hospital, family, close friends). Post pregnancy, it is also very important that you arrange time for yourself and time alone with your partner if you are in a relationship. We will discuss this in more detail, but it helps life stay calm and will help you feel more in control.

- **Competency and achievement**: Feeling proud of ourselves, feeling 'good enough', is very important to our emotional well-being. In today's fast-paced society, we are measured against others in many ways, so feeling inadequate has unfortunately become commonplace, especially amongst mothers. We will discuss this in more depth later on.

- **Attention**: Giving and receiving attention is essential to normal development and emotional well-being. Everyone needs a sense of inclusion and appreciation, to feel their presence has been noted. During and after pregnancy, this need is often compromised. We must not lose sight of the fact that we matter, we deserve attention.

- **Connection to others**: Our brains are social organs. In the womb, neurons in the developing brain become functional only if they connect with other neurons, implying that it is in our make-up to interact and be part of something. Pregnancy can make it difficult to stay in touch with others, but it very important to stay involved with other adults. Make a point of meeting friends and staying connected.

- **Purpose and meaning:** This comes from being creative and challenged. Countless studies have shown that having a strong sense of purpose in life is associated with greater overall mental health, happiness and even longevity. Having a baby gives a huge sense of purpose, but we can have other purposes too: things that stretch our minds or bodies, things we can look forward to doing. These could be anything from taking classes to learning something new at home.

- **Fun and relaxation**: Life without fun and relaxation can easily become meaningless. The human mind and body cannot go through life on a constant flow of adrenaline. We must have down time, time to relax and have fun. Play with your baby, have a laugh with those around you, take time out. You will feel the benefit of it, I promise!

- **Love and affection**: Everyone needs to feel loved and cared for, whether by a partner or by someone else. I guess it's the world's way of saying we are worthwhile. Love is the basis of every creation.

- **Your relationship:** If you are in a relationship, it is important that you nurture it during and after pregnancy. A new baby has a big impact on 'couple life', so adjustments might need to be made to ensure that the sparkle between you and your partner stays bright. Researchers at the Murdoch Childrens Research Institute in Victoria, Australia, interviewed 1,500 new mothers about intimacy and sexual health as part of a longitudinal study. They found that:

> Lifestyle changes associated with having a baby, loss of freedom and loss of time together as a couple are challenges for all new parents and can be overwhelming at times . . . For some women, motherhood and sexuality are experienced as contradictory roles.

Most women said they had sex less often, even after twelve months, than they had before they became pregnant, with intimacy taking a back seat to the love and energy being poured into their newborn. Thankfully, if you are conscious of this and nurture your relationship, having a baby only makes your love all the more wonderful. Here are some tips to help you:

- The most important thing in any relationship is communication. If you keep talking and being honest, you'll keep that strong bond.

- Coordinate a schedule with your partner regarding who cares for the baby, especially at night. If possible, alternate feedings so that each parent can get a chunk of uninterrupted sleep. Until your child is sleeping for longer stretches at night, coordinating a schedule so that each parent can get a nap will be beneficial as well. It prevents sleep deprivation irritability.

- After a baby is born, there is a normal lull in sexual activity. Keep the relationship strong by cuddling up together, holding hands and kissing.

- Accept your partner's initiation of affection as sign of their love for you.

- When you have family members available to babysit, take advantage of this and put a date night on the calendar! Schedule date nights in advance.

- Talk about things other than your baby sometimes.

- Point out the things your partner is doing well. We all have different ways of doing things, but make sure you encourage your partner by pointing out the positive things. Sending a text with these small affirmations is also a great way to build your connection as parents.

- **Feeling attractive**: Although not a vital human need, for most people – and especially for women – it is important. During pregnancy, we might wonder if our baby bump puts our partner off. It doesn't! In fact, studies show that most men find their partner's pregnancy bump very beautiful. Post pregnancy, we might question if our partner finds us attractive. It takes time for the pregnancy bump to go down, your boobs may look a bit on the ready-to-explode side, especially if you are nursing, and the *linea nigra* (the brown pregnancy line that runs from your navel to the pubic area) takes time to disappear. It's a natural concern but not something our partners concern themselves with. I know it's hard to believe, since we can feel so frumpy, but the fact is, it's not up to us to decide what our partners should think. Their thoughts are theirs to have, not ours.

Balance or Imbalance?

Now it's time to rate your current situation. I'd like you to shade in each area of the wheel on the facing page, which will graphically represent how balanced your needs are on a scale of one to ten. A score of one is the innermost point and ten is the outer edge of the circle. If you feel a need is totally balanced, it would score a ten. If a need is totally imbalanced, it would score a one. And if a need is average, it would score a five, and so on. We want a graphic representation of what your life looks like right now so we can measure your progress.

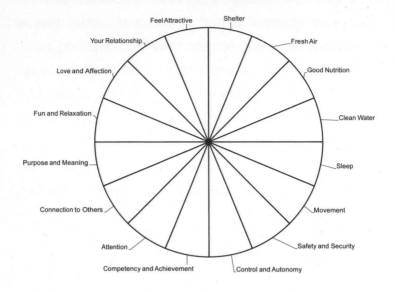

How did you score? Relax! As I said, most people's needs are imbalanced. But imagine for a moment putting that wheel on your car and taking a drive. How rough do you think it would feel – pretty bumpy, right? Life is the same. Might this explain why you have not been feeling or looking as amazing as you want to?

Your First Step

In the spaces below, write one step you can take to get each of your needs more in balance *today*. I will help you with this throughout the book but, for now, write down a simple step you can implement today to make a difference, no matter how small. For example, you might take a little walk, drink an extra glass of water, give yourself a half an hour of quiet time or maybe meet a friend. Whatever it is, write it down.

Physical Needs

Shelter

_____

_____

_____

_____

_____

_____

_____

_____

Fresh Air

_____

_____

_____

_____

_____

_____

_____

_____

Good nutrition

_____

_____

_____

_____

_____

_____

_____

Clean Water

_____

_____

_____

_____

_____

_____

Sleep

_____

_____

_____

_____

_____

_____

Movement

_____

_____

_____

_____

_____

_____

_____

Emotional Needs

Safety and Security

_____

_____

_____

_____

_____

_____

_____

Control and Autonomy

_____

_____

_____

_____

_____

Competency and Achievement

_____

_____

_____

_____

_____

_____

_____

Attention

_____

_____

_____

_____

_____

_____

_____

Connection to Others

_____

_____

_____

_____

_____

_____

_____

Purpose and Meaning

_____

_____

_____

_____

_____

_____

_____

Fun and Relaxation

_____

_____

_____

_____

_____

_____

_____

Love and Affection

_____

_____

_____

_____

_____

_____

_____

_____

Your Relationship

_____

_____

_____

_____

_____

_____

_____

Feeling Attractive

_____

_____

_____

_____

_____

_____

_____

Putting You in a Position for Maintainable Results!

By identifying, rating and improving upon your needs you put yourself in a very strong position for implementing the _Born to Be Beautiful_ plan. No matter how balanced or imbalanced your needs are at the moment, by being conscious of them you can improve your situation each day, laying a strong foundation for looking and feeling amazing. This foundation will allow you to maintain your results long-term, not just for a few days or weeks. For example, let's say we find ourselves comfort-eating, perhaps out of loneliness or boredom. We could work on making sure we have better connections with others and more time with our partners, filling the need gap, so to speak. Another example: if we find ourselves overtired, maybe we need to work on getting more rest. It's a matter of identifying what's imbalanced and correcting it so your needs are met correctly. Take a small step each day, every day. If you make just a one percent improvement each day, which is doable, at the end of the year you will be 365 percent better than you are now!

Tell People What You Need

It can be quite frustrating when other people don't understand or notice that we need something, especially when the people are those who are supposed to love us. But the truth is it's not their job to make our lives better, although it would be nice if that were the case. If you need something then ask for it, do not wait for it to be given.

People love you but they have their own lives. They may not even notice that there is something you need. It doesn't mean they don't care, it may simply mean that they didn't realise you needed it or it may not be something that would matter to them personally, and that is okay. Everyone has different values and things that matter to them. Sometimes people just don't know what's going on. Even if we would like them to be mind readers, they are not, so if you want help or need change, verbalise it. Now, when you do that, don't automatically expect a positive response (if you get it, great). Verbalising what you need simply makes it easier for everyone. It clarifies the situation so if you don't get the response you had hoped for you can look for an appropriate, alternative way of getting your needs met.

You cannot be all things to all people all of the time. We all need a bit of help now and then. Be gentle and kind to yourself.

2
You and Your Goal

The Supermom

When you become a mother, it is so easy to put pressure on yourself to be Supermom, expecting yourself to do everything right all of the time and look good in the process. It's a huge burden to carry, especially considering the Supermom concept is just an illusion of perfection. I know, because I was considered a Supermom. Some people thought I just floated through pregnancy without any hiccups and that I have done everything effortlessly since. The reality is very different. I needed help both physically and emotionally during my pregnancy. I had seizures, which made things quite difficult. When it was time to give birth to my baby, I struggled through sixteen hours of labour, wailed like a scraggly haired lunatic throughout (not a pretty sight!) and gave birth balling my eyes out and exhausted. Since then, every day I change my baby's smelly nappies, I clean his dirty, snotty face and I play toy pick-up with him fifty times a day, just the same as every other mom. Unless you have a full-time superhuman step-in, it's one-size fits all – motherhood is motherhood.

I got my figure back and I felt amazing not because of being better than anyone else, but solely by implementing the *Born to Be Beautiful* plan every day and asking for help if and when I needed it.

I designed the plan for a mom who can't do everything all the time, because when I was pregnant, I couldn't. I needed something that I could do comfortably at home and that fitted in with my life. And now, having given birth to my baby, I do most things with him by my side. I have to work around him or with him, so this is very much a workable plan. The plan was designed for real life, for you.

Be Authentic!

I want you to be authentic and true to yourself and your baby. Don't get caught up in silly illusions of perfection that ultimately make us miserable. This book is not intended to help you be like somebody else or create a more convincing facade to try to impress the world. Instead, it will bring you more in touch with your authentic self and fill you with the energy to be the best *you* can be, to be the best version of *yourself*. It will give you the opportunity to allow your body to perform at its best and to develop your mind so you feel amazing every day.

In one way or another, every day we are bombarded by messages that we should be better, that we are not good enough. But good enough compared to whom? Who defined what good enough means? Marketing companies, that's who, companies that know how to play with our egos for profit. It has been drilled into us that we should be someone else's version of perfection. If we are short we want to be tall, if we have straight hair we want curly hair, if we have light-coloured hair we want dark-coloured hair. The fact is you are already good enough! You are absolutely unique and so you cannot be compared to anyone else. Even if you have a twin, you are unique. There is not a single person on the planet the same as you, which makes you very special indeed. Besides, you can only ever be second-rate to somebody else, but you can always be first-rate to you.

Your Mind, Conditioned

Imagine this scenario: I bring you to a computer store to buy a new laptop. As we are browsing, a sales assistant approaches us and asks us if we would like some help. We accept. He goes on to explain which one he thinks we should buy. Let's say we are not knowledgeable about computers and we opt for the laptop he recommends. Picking it off the shelf, he asks if we want some extra programmes so we can do many things on the laptop. Again, not knowing much about the products, we trust his judgment and buy the ones he recommends. After all, he is the expert.

A little while later, we decide to test out what we've bought. We turn on the laptop and, by following instructions, we install the programmes. Feeling accomplished, we proceed to play around with the programmes. It's tricky at first but, after an hour, we learn how to navigate our way around. Over the next few months, using the laptop every day, we become very good at using the programmes. A year later, we can operate the programmes as easily as we can turn on a TV.

Now I want you to liken that laptop experience to your brain. Just like we went into the computer store, when we are born we are brought into the world. Instead of getting a laptop, we get a brain. Instead of computer programmes surrounding us, we get information from other people and things. The sales assistant could be likened to the people we meet in life, the people who were born into the world long before us. Just as we trusted the sales assistant's recommendations, we trust the 'experts' around us. After all, they have been here longer than us so they are more knowledgeable. We accept what they say, we mimic what they do and we follow their instructions. With regular practice, over time we become good at what we learn. For example, I was brought into the world in an English-speaking family and, not surprisingly, I learned to speak English. My friend, on the other hand, was born into a French-speaking family. Guess what she speaks? We learn what we are exposed to.

Since being born, we have received programmes/information every second. Some of the programmes are useful and some are not. Unfortunately, just as a laptop cannot tell how useful a programme is, our brains accept whatever they are given, good or bad. And just as a bad programme installed on a laptop causes frustration when it doesn't operate properly, we find ourselves frustrated when we don't operate effectively. We get upset when things don't turn out the way we want or when we behave in ways we don't like. Everything we do is an imitation of or a response to something we picked up along the way – everything from our accent and language to our state of mind and physical health.

Having said that, the fact that we have been programmed is not an excuse for how our lives are now. You accepted the junk you were fed, just as a laptop would accept junk mail. No matter who said or did what, ultimately we are responsible for how our lives turn out from now onwards. It's time to take ownership of the results you want in your life from *now* on. If you want to feel and look amazing you must be prepared to put aside the thoughts and behaviours that don't serve you and let go of the past. Fortunately, modern science has made the process easier for us.

For years, scientists have talked about how complex the human brain is but, as more research is conducted, it seems we operate on very simple, mechanical systems, so it's much easier to programme (and reprogramme) ourselves than was once thought. Using MRI scans and electroencephalograms, we are now able to see how our brains behave in various situations: how they accept, deal with and change information. Our brains can do many things, which might make them seem complex, but the reality is that they operate from very simplistic systems – many systems, but simplistic ones nonetheless. We can see how they respond to various stimuli and what parts activate for what reasons.

The Limbic System

We now know that most of our environmental programming takes place in an area of the brain called the limbic system. This part of our brain is quite primitive (all animals have it) and is also responsible for our emotional associations and responses. This would explain why certain songs or smells evoke certain emotions in us. For example, if we experience a certain song on vacation or at a funeral, whatever emotion we experienced at the time will be attached to the song. When the song is played in the future, the same emotions will be triggered almost instantly – a classic example of programming in action.

Studies have shown that the limbic system also finds it very difficult, on a neurological level, to tell the difference between reality and imagination. It has been found that the brain engages the same neurological reactions, whether we are doing something for real or merely imagining doing it. These patterns are similar to small tracks engraved in the brain cells. So, if at some point in time we associated an intense emotion with a situation, stimulus or behaviour, as soon as we come in contact with the same – or a similar – situation, stimulus or behaviour, the same emotions will be triggered. This is one reason why we avoid doing things that on a logical level would benefit us, such as practising things that we want to become confident in.

Example: Jane found social interaction very difficult. She felt comfortable in one-to-one situations but when it came to group situations she felt terrified. As a result, she became shy and avoided situations where she might find herself in groups, such as parties and events.

Why did she feel this way? Aren't groups just a bunch of individuals bunched together? It's not as if when an individual joins four others they change or become dangerous. The limbic system doesn't operate from logic, though. It operates from emotionally tagged programmes. You see, six years earlier, Jane had been bullied by a group at work. She feared the same painful experience happening again. Although she wanted to attend parties and events, her emotionally tagged programme wouldn't let her, in the event it brought her pain again. It was only when she let go of the emotions associated with the bullying at work that she could go on to feel comfortable in groups.

Programming and associations happen at a neurological level and because our brains operate at lightning speed we often don't consciously know why we do what we do. But there are so many reasons for why we do what we do. For some it's being told they we're stupid at school. For others, it may be a brief comment about height, hair, voice or ability. For others it's simply a matter of repeating a behaviour so often that it becomes a habit. You could drive yourself mad trying to figure it out. You already know how you feel and look; analysing it will not change it. Fortunately, you don't need to figure it out to change or drop the programme. You simply need to reprogramme your brain for successful results and good feelings.

Reprogramming

Top athletes are known to use a process called visualisation as part of their training sessions. Not only does it create focus, it is also used to create a renewed and heightened sense of well-being and confidence. Visualisation is sometimes referred to as guided imagery, mental rehearsal or mediation, but the basic techniques and concepts are the same. Generally speaking, visualisation is the process of creating a mental image or intention of what you want to feel or to have happen. Athletes use this technique to achieve a specific outcome in a race or training session. By imagining a previous best performance or a future, desired performance, the athlete becomes part of the feeling associated with the achievement. These imagined scenarios can include any of the senses. They can be visual (images of crossing the finish line), kinaesthetic (sensations of winning) or auditory (sounds of a crowd cheering). By using their mind, an athlete can call up these images again and again, enhancing the skill through repetition or rehearsal. Such repeated imagery has been shown to strengthen neural responses in the brain and is used to build confidence in an athlete's ability to perform certain skills under pressure.

Fortunately for us, we don't have to be athletes to use this process to get desired results. We can use the same process to enhance our physiques and emotional well-being as moms. I used this technique often during my pregnancy and I still use it. For example, I would imagine my tummy tightening and looking its best. Our brains naturally send messages via neural pathways to make this happen in reality.

Don't believe me? Try it now for yourself. Close your eyes and imagine your tummy tightening and you looking and feeling exactly as you want. You might find that even as I ask you to imagine it, you feel your tummy muscles start to contract automatically. If not, they will when you do the exercise with purpose. You see, when it comes to our neural responses and training our minds and bodies, our brains do it at a cellular level and, at that level, they find it very difficult to differentiate between what we are simply rehearsing in our minds and what we are doing in reality.

We can be aware of what we are doing consciously but, on a cellular level, our brains are working away in the background, doing what needs to be done to get a result. Your brain is responsible for your heart beating, your body functioning, your memories resurfacing and so much more. Your unconscious mind is working for you all of the time. You can literally train it to help you look and feel amazing.

So, once you have identified your personal goal within the *Born to Be Beautiful* plan, I would like you to rehearse your positive physical and emotional outcomes in your mind over and over in detail, with emotion, before it even comes to fruition. It will encourage your brain to immediately set up the necessary neural pathways. You can strengthen your responses with the daily purposeful actions that I will show you in the following chapters. We're going to get very specific about what you need to do.

Set Your Goals

Research has shown time and again that people who set and write down goals are more likely to achieve them than people who don't, and to achieve them more quickly. Writing down our goals allows for additional neural strengthening. I would like you now to write down your physical goal and your emotional goal. We will break these down shortly, but for now just outline your bigger picture, your ultimate result.

Write down how you want to look post pregnancy. Write it in as much detail as possible so you can really get a sense of what you want. How would you look and physically feel at your body's healthiest? Do you want to have a certain level of tone or fitness? Do you want a flat, stretch-mark-free tummy? What clothes will you wear? How would you like your hair to look? In your mind, see how people respond positively to you. Write it all down in detail and add a picture if you like. Make sure to state it in the positive form for maximum effectiveness. For example, instead of saying 'I don't want to be fat,' say 'I will be healthy, slim and toned.' Whatever your goals are, write them down now.

_____

_____

_____

_____

_____

_____

_____

_____

_____

_____

_____

_____

_____

_____

_____

_____

Now write down how you want to feel post pregnancy. Do you want to feel confident? Loving? Accomplished? Caring? Outgoing? Calm? Write in detail how you want to feel, and see yourself feeling that way. Again, state it in the positive form. Instead of writing 'I don't want to be shy anymore,' put 'I will be confident and proud to be the best me I can be.'

_____

_____

_____

_____

_____

_____

_____

_____

_____

_____

_____

_____

_____

_____

_____

_____

_____

Give Your Brain a Reason

Having a good reason to achieve a goal is important – I would go so far as to say essential. It's very difficult to maintain anything if we put no purpose behind it. Think about it: how much more quickly and easily do people get in shape if they have a wedding or vacation coming up? How much more quickly do people gain confidence when they have a speech to give? We do things when we have a reason to do them. So, you must now ask yourself *why* you want to look and feel amazing. Why is it important to you? What will it mean for you and those around you?

_____
_____
_____
_____
_____
_____
_____
_____
_____
_____
_____
_____
_____
_____
_____
_____
_____
_____
_____

The Benefits

Our brains get most excited and active when we generate an emotional or physical association with something. How quickly do you learn not to put your hand on a hot plate – super fast, right? That is because your brain has a strong association with heat. How quickly does a song evoke emotion if it is associated with someone we love – lightning speed? So, to get you results fast, we need to create some positive tags to achieving your goals. I would like you to list the benefits of looking and feeling your best. What good things will it do for you? What good things will it do for your baby? What good things will it do for the people around you? This is very important and will help you maintain results long-term. When your brain realises that looking and feeling amazing will also benefit others, it will be easier to achieve what you want. Your brain will want to do it!

_____

_____

_____

_____

_____

_____

_____

_____

_____

_____

_____

_____

_____

_____

_____

_____

_____

Strengths and Resources

Now that your brain has a 'why' and can see the benefits of implementing the *Born to Be Beautiful* plan, it is a good idea to acknowledge that sometimes life gets in the way of what we want to achieve and we feel like giving up. Everything can be going great and then life can throw a spanner in the works that causes our motivation to dwindle and eventually fade out altogether.

That *won't* be happening here! I'm very aware that life can pose challenges, so we are preparing ourselves for that possibility in advance of setting your goal. There may be times where you feel extra-challenged or, for whatever reason, something gets in the way of you implementing the *Born to Be Beautiful* plan fully, but reminding yourself that you have strengths and resources to draw upon if you need them at any stage throughout the plan can make things much easier. There have undoubtedly been challenges in your life that, at the time, seemed insurmountable, but that you managed to deal with by drawing on your resources and strengths. In hindsight, if you knew you would deal with them so well *in advance* of having to deal with them, you wouldn't have stressed out half as much, right?

Strengths might be personal characteristics or abilities. Resources could be anything from friends to family to finances. Anything you can draw upon should you need it could be a strength or a resource. Please write your strengths and resources on the lines below.

_____

_____

_____

_____

_____

_____

_____

_____

_____

_____

_____

_____

_____

_____

Set Your Stepping Stones

The best way to achieve a goal is to set out exactly what must be done and when. This allows us to track and measure progress. We are going to use an eighteen-month time frame, although you are likely to achieve your desired outcome much faster using the *Born to Be Beautiful* plan. In the space below, outline where you want to be eighteen months post pregnancy (or from now if you've already had your baby). Having this written down clearly and referring to it often will allow you to focus more easily.

18-Month Goal

Now I want you to ask yourself where you will need to be at each stage indicated below, if you are to achieve your eighteen-month goal. For example, in the first section, under twelve months, you will write where you will need to be in twelve months if you are to achieve your eighteen-month goal. In the next section, under six months, you will write where you will need to be in six months if you are to achieve your twelve-month goal, and so on. You will fill out the majority of this when you finish this book – after you get to the nitty-gritty action steps! – to make sure you implement the exact steps you'll need to take in order to look and feel amazing during and after pregnancy. For now, just fill in your targets as you see them. It is *essential* that you complete these sections, so I have included them again (with action steps) in the final chapter. This will be your guide over the next eighteen months.

12-Month Goal

_____
_____
_____
_____
_____
_____
_____

_____

_____

_____

_____

_____

_____

6-Month Goal

_____

_____

_____

_____

_____

_____

_____

_____

_____

_____

3-Month Goal

_____

_____

_____

_____

_____

_____

_____

_____

_____

_____

_____

_____

1-Month Goal

_____

_____

_____

_____

_____

_____

_____

_____

_____

_____

_____

_____

_____

1-Week Goal

_____

_____

_____

_____

_____

_____

_____

_____

_____

_____

_____

Today's Goal

_____

_____

_____

_____

_____

_____

_____

_____

_____

_____

_____

_____

_____

_____

_____

Referring to these goals on a regular basis will help keep you focused. A good way to do this is to tick off your daily and weekly goals as you achieve them. This will allow you to do everything in small, manageable steps. You will be able to measure your progress and feel a sense of accomplishment as you see yourself reaching your targets. Keep your action steps simple, small and consistent, and the bigger goal will take care of itself.

Reward Yourself for Reaching Targets

'Recognise and reward the good' has become commonplace teaching in developmental and educational psychology. When a child says his or her first word, we celebrate. When they stand for the first time, we celebrate. When they get their first gold star at school, we celebrate. It is just so natural and beautiful to celebrate a triumph in a child's life. And you are in fact just a grown-up child. There is no point in a book of life that says the celebration must stop at a certain age. It's all just conditioning. So celebrate achieving targets and celebrate often!

You Can Do This!

Implementing a plan during and after pregnancy may seem daunting. There was a time during my pregnancy when I totally lacked motivation. Everything was going great and then, all of a sudden, I just couldn't be bothered. Not being able to move about as fast I'd like (I was a busy bee before I became pregnant) and getting so big that the only thing I could wear was leggings really got to me. I hate leggings! With each day, I felt dowdier than the previous one, not because I looked bad but because I felt I was losing my identity in a way. I couldn't help but see myself at home with a child on my hip, big granny bows in my hair, sweating over a pot of soup like the old woman in the shoe. And then there were times when I felt too tired to even care what was happening. Post pregnancy was the same. My goal was there but occasionally tiredness poked its head up, waiting to be used as an excuse for me to give up the plan. Thankfully, I didn't give in.

If at any time you feel your enthusiasm dipping, just acknowledge the feeling as normal (we all have off days) and let it go. Hear these words in your mind: 'I can look and feel amazing! Stay focused.' Write it on an affirmation card if you'd like, and hang it somewhere you will see it often. In the final chapter, we will discuss how you can create and maintain momentum. Now it is time to look at what you can expect and learn the specific action steps you'll need to take so you look and feel amazing.

3
What to Expect

Pregnancy brings with it lots of changes, everything from mood swings to a swollen tummy, from sausage fingers to loose teeth. The key to controlling what happens *after* pregnancy is understanding *how* your body and mood change during pregnancy and working *with* nature, not against it, so you achieve the results you want. We will look at what physical and emotional changes you can expect during and after pregnancy. It will allow you to see that certain changes are absolutely normal (and essential), and it will help you to avoid the things that aren't normal or that you don't want. Most importantly, you will know exactly what to do to ensure you get all the things you do want!

Weight Gain

Weight gain is perhaps one of the top issues women struggle with when they become pregnant. It can cause a lot of emotional upset, so we will look at it first. Although it may be difficult to accept, weight gain is an essential *temporary* change. You must gain a certain amount of weight during pregnancy if you and your baby are to be healthy. It is normal and necessary. By implementing what I show you, you will be able to stay within guidelines during pregnancy and enjoy an amazing physique post pregnancy.

The average woman will gain anywhere from twenty pounds to thirty-five pounds during pregnancy. During the conception period, the uterus can expand to one thousand times its original size. During pregnancy, the placenta grows, amniotic fluid surrounds your baby and your body holds fifty percent more blood than it did before pregnancy, amongst other changes. If your body was to remain the same weight with all this in place, it would be very unhealthy. Being too skinny during pregnancy is *not* the way to go. If you don't put on what we will call *good pregnancy weight*, you are at a higher risk of delivering a preterm baby or a low-birth-weight baby, which can be dangerous.

Having said that, a need to gain a certain amount of weight in pregnancy does not mean you get an automatic license to eat the fridge empty. Common sense will tell you that. Contrary to what you may have heard, you are not eating for two – at least not two adults. A growing baby does not need adult calorie intake. In fact, you only need an extra three hundred calories for your baby's healthy growth. That's equivalent to a cup of cereal, eight ounces of milk and a banana. Our aim here is balance. In the event that you have already put on extra weight (exceeding the guidelines), or if you're reading this post pregnancy, there's no need to panic. I will show you healthy ways of dealing with weight gain.

Good Pregnancy Weight

There are two aspects to consider when deciding what normal, healthy weight gain is for you. The first is your pre-pregnancy weight, and the second is the composition of inevitable, internal changes. Your doctor will weigh you when your pregnancy is confirmed and several times throughout your pregnancy to make sure you are gaining enough weight. The following are general guidelines for you to work with.

Pre-pregnancy Weight

- If your pre-pregnancy weight is within the healthy range for your height, you should gain between twenty-five and thirty-five pounds.

- If you are underweight for your height, you should gain twenty-eight to forty pounds.

- If you are overweight for your height, you should gain fifteen to twenty-five pounds.

- If you are obese, you should gain between eleven and twenty pounds.

- If you're having twins, you should gain thirty-seven to fifty-four pounds if you start at a healthy weight, thirty-one to fifty pounds if you are overweight and twenty-five to forty-two pounds if you are obese.

Weight Composition

The weight you gain should be pregnancy weight, not unnecessary fat. The following are guidelines for the approximate composition of pregnancy weight.

- Baby: eight pounds

- Placenta: two to three pounds

- Amniotic fluid: two to three pounds

- Breast tissue: two to three pounds

- Blood supply: four pounds

- Stored fat for delivery and breastfeeding: five to nine pounds

- Larger uterus: two to five pounds

Cravings

Not all women get cravings during pregnancy but it's very common. Some cravings even extend beyond pregnancy. When I was pregnant, I had an insatiable craving for crushed ice with a bit of pineapple juice on top. I know it sounds crazy! But the strangest thing is that I hated ice before pregnancy – even the crunch of it sent shivers up my spine – but during pregnancy I couldn't get enough of it. Morning, noon and night I had to have my crushed ice with juice on top. If I couldn't get it I felt irritable, sometimes angry. It would be safe to say that I would easily have licked the ice off a freezer shelf. Seriously, it was that bad. Thankfully, I never had to. I made sure to always have trays of ice ready! A friend of mine had an equally strong craving. She couldn't get enough salty and spicy food. Spicy and greasy takeouts, chips laden with salt and vinegar, and *dilsk* (seaweed) – she was totally addicted. Some women even crave things like coal or soap. How crazy is that? What part of the mind overrides logic to say it's okay to crave coal or soap? But when you have a craving, it feels like you'll nearly die if you don't get what you feel you need. Logic doesn't come into it at all. You know you shouldn't eat something, yet it's so hard not to. It is incredibly frustrating and, if it's junk food, it can make staying within guidelines very difficult.

The Secret Behind Cravings

Thankfully, pregnancy cravings are not just batty thoughts. They are not out of our control. With the right information, we can counteract them. They are often caused by an imbalance in the body, an unmet need! I was totally baffled by my craving. It didn't make any sense to me whatsoever so I decided to do some research and find out if I could do anything to stop it.

After a bit of research, I came to the conclusion that I wasn't turning into an Inuit; instead, there was a strong possibility that I had low iron levels in my blood. Of course, ice and iron deficiency seemed to be an odd match, but I decided to get checked anyway. Lo and behold, a quick blood test at the hospital confirmed that my iron levels were low. I increased my iron intake and the craving dissipated within a few days.

Something so simple yet, without the awareness and correction, it had been driving me mad. The interesting thing is, when I was doing my research I discovered that other cravings are usually due to mineral deficiencies also. Chocolate, greasy food, spices, soda, salt, etc. – they can all just be mineral deficiencies that can easily be sorted out. I was lucky, ice isn't fattening, but can you imagine if I had had cravings for chocolate or candy? I'm sure I would have found them very difficult to resist, which could have resulted in totally unnecessary weight gain.

Cravings can be managed. If you find yourself unable to stop eating certain foods, get your blood checked before you have a go at yourself for being weak or indulgent. If there is a deficiency, it's simply a matter of balancing the mineral or vitamin as recommended by your doctor. Overproduction of a hormone called prolactin can cause cravings, as can dehydration.

During pregnancy, the placenta secretes prolactin. Although it's a useful chemical (it helps reduce anxiety and pain) and a necessary one (it leads to the production of breast milk) it can be overproduced and it can activate the elements of the brain associated with addictive behaviour. Yes, prolactin is the other culprit for the munchies. Not only that, it is responsible for a slow-down in fat metabolism, with resulting unnecessary weight gain. But fear not, it can be managed. Studies show that there's a link between overproduction of prolactin and vitamin B6 deficiency, so simply consider eating more foods containing vitamin B6, such as potatoes, bananas and spinach. Even if you don't know if a craving is due to prolactin overload, eat foods rich in B6 anyway. They are good for you and will help your baby. Another study showed that zinc can decrease prolactin levels, so consider eating foods high in zinc also. Shellfish, turkey and beans have good zinc content.

During pregnancy, it's very easy to become dehydrated. Your doctor will no doubt tell you that you need to drink more water during pregnancy but when you're not conscious of it day to day, it is very easy to forget to drink enough. You can suddenly feel parched and not know why, but if you are thirsty it is an indication that you are dehydrated, not just becoming so. What most people don't know is that thirst and hunger signals (weakness, a grumbling stomach, etc.) are controlled by the same part of your brain, namely the hypothalamus. The hypothalamus helps your nervous system communicate with your endocrine system, which includes your organs, glands and hormones. When your stomach is empty, specific hormones are released to signal hunger. The hypothalamus receives these signals and tells the nervous system that it's time to eat when, really, it could be time to drink water. In light of this, if you find that you are hungry but you know you've eaten only a short time ago, chances are you are dehydrated and a good drink of water will sort the problem out. And if you drink water before meals, as a rule, you will not only stay hydrated throughout the day, you will trick your brain into feeling fuller quicker. This also applies post pregnancy.

Structural Changes

It is inevitable that you will also experience structural changes in your body during pregnancy. It is not a bad thing. They are changes that have to happen to allow for the healthy growth of your baby. Go with the flow, listen to your body and embrace the fact that structural changes will happen and are perfectly fine. The important thing to know is how to prevent unwanted damage following the changes, such as marks and sagging skin. This is where you must put certain things in place to help nature steer itself in the right direction or reverse damage if it's already been done. Later in the book we will discuss in detail how to prevent stretch marks and sagging skin but for now let's get an initial overview of what you can expect to happen in the areas of your body that are affected by the pregnancy experience.

Tummy

To accommodate your growing baby and the extra weight you gain during pregnancy, your body softens your ligaments so your pelvis can open to allow the safe passage of the baby's head. Postural changes will follow and these can cause your tummy muscles to stretch and become weak. Your rib cage and diaphragm also need to budge out of the way to allow for your baby's healthy growth. Combined with the effects of yo-yoing hormones, these structural changes can lead to a condition called *diastasis recti*, which is basically a separation of the abdominal muscles. Many women don't even know they have *diastasis recti*, although back pain is an indication. You will learn in this book how *diastasis recti* can be managed so you can have your sexy tummy post pregnancy.

Boobs

Oh yes, the boob sprout. For ladies on the small side, the sudden growth is a godsend. However, for those more endowed, it can be a nightmare to search for a bra that fits. Either way, the growth is not due to fat – it is caused by swollen milk glands. Your boobs will continue to grow throughout your pregnancy, but after you deliver and finish nursing, they will return to their pre-pregnancy size or possibly smaller. In order to make sure your boobs look great after pregnancy it's essential that you wear a supportive bra throughout your pregnancy. Without support, the extra weight is going to strain the connective tissues, which can lead to sagging and overstretching which, in turn, can lead to stretch marks. Doing pectoral exercises can help strengthen the muscles under your breasts, something you will learn about in Chapter 6.

Skin Changes

When you are pregnant your skin needs to stretch to accommodate your growing bump and your newfound milk machines. Since I was carrying a big baby, my bump was huge and my skin stretched to the point where it felt like it was going to tear open. For the purposes of this book, it is important that we put measures in place to prevent your skin tearing. Your skin must be elastic enough to accommodate pregnancy growth and bounce back into shape post pregnancy. What we want to do is make sure your skin behaves itself and does what we want it to do when we need it to. Skin changes are going to happen, everything from stretching to changes in colour. Even oil production can be affected. But once we know that, we can naturally manipulate it to work in our favour.

Elastin and Collagen

Elastin is a protein in connective tissue that is elastic and helps skin to return to its original position when it's poked or pinched. Enough elastin in the skin means that the skin will bounce back to its normal shape after a pull. It keeps the skin smooth as it stretches to accommodate normal activities like flexing a muscle or opening and closing the mouth. As you grow during pregnancy you want to make sure that your skin has the maximum possible stretching capacity. Damage to elastic tissue can't be avoided and is part of the natural aging process. The aim here is to protect our elastin as best we can.

Elastin is often an ingredient in 'anti-aging' products and moisturisers, but did you know that these proteins do not and cannot penetrate the skin, which they would have to if they were going to make it more elastic? I am sorry to tell you that you have being spending your hard-earned cash on lotions and potions that don't even penetrate your skin. They can form a temporary coating on the skin, and that helps the skin hold in moisture, but they will not provide more flexibility or inject moisture into the skin itself. In fact, elastin skin care products have been shown to have little effect on skin elasticity at all. Not only that, elastin works in conjunction with collagen (a natural firming protein) but products containing collagen have very little effect either, despite what skin-care companies claim. It cannot be absorbed from the outside; it must be produced internally.

As someone who didn't want to get sagging skin or stretch marks, I asked myself how elastin and collagen are naturally produced in the body, especially during pregnancy, and I aimed to protect the elastin and collagen I had. Elastin is made up of amino acids, which are the building blocks of protein, so I made sure to eat the correct proteins throughout my pregnancy. I cannot say for sure if eating these specific proteins contributed to my skin not sagging but my skin didn't sag so it's worth eating the right proteins if you're eating proteins anyway. The amino acids that make up elastin are: glycine, alanine, valine and proline. Glycine, alanine and proline are produced by the body naturally but valine is not. I made sure to eat foods containing valine. Good food sources of valine include egg whites (make sure they are properly cooked), soy protein, spirulina, seaweed and fish. Stock up on valine-rich foods.

There are also foods that are said to be linked to collagen growth. The six foods I made sure to eat were: garlic, soy protein, tomatoes, omega-3 fatty acids (found in oily fish and chia seeds), dark green vegetables and red-coloured fruit. All contain components that are said to promote collagen growth. Again, I cannot say for sure that eating these foods protected my elastin and collagen but, reflecting on my research and my own results, I would encourage you to eat them as they may well be an important factor in keeping a firm body.

Redness, a.k.a. 'The Pregnancy Glow'

When a person gets embarrassed, blood rushes to the surface of their skin, causing redness. Something similar happens in pregnancy: During pregnancy, your body produces fifty percent more blood than normal. The extra blood, together with the temperature increase pregnancy brings, makes your skin appear redder.

Tip: Dab your face with rose water and witch hazel. You can get these in health stores. Both have toning, calming effects. They will not rid the problem entirely, but they will help. They also remove excess oil from skin, so you will avoid the shiny, red ball look.

Pimples and Acne

During pregnancy, the extra hormones in your body cause your oil glands to secrete more oil, which can cause breakouts. If you have a problem with acne already, your acne may become worse for a while.

Tip: Clean your face properly day and night using tea tree oil diluted in water, which also has antibacterial benefits. You can get tea tree oil in health stores. After cleansing, remove any excess oil with witch hazel or rose water, using a cotton pad, then smear a thin layer of pure aloe vera gel on your face.

Dark, Splotchy Patches

Nearly fifty percent of pregnant women show some signs of dark, splotches during pregnancy.

Pregnancy-related hormones can cause an increase in skin pigmentation.

Tip: To avoid post pregnancy damage, make sure you avoid direct sunlight during pregnancy. That means no sunbathing and the use of sun cream with SPF 30+.

Varicose Veins

Varicose veins are bulky, bluish veins that usually appear on the legs during pregnancy. This happens because your body is compensating for the extra blood flow that is going to your baby. If you have a family history of varicose veins, which I do, you may be prone to getting them during your pregnancy. They can be avoided.

Tips:

- Move! You need to get your blood flowing so it gets to your heart.

- Put your feet up for at least a half an hour a day. Prop them up with a cushion or lie on the floor with your feet on the wall.

- Don't cross your legs when sitting and don't sit for long periods of time.

- Add witch hazel to a moisturiser and rub it into your legs. It strengthens vein walls, which improves circulation and helps to prevent varicose and spider veins from forming. Witch hazel also closes swollen veins, making them less visible.

- Wear support stockings (under trousers so that you don't frighten people), especially when travelling. They look awful but it's worth it.

- Get enough vitamin C, which helps keep your veins healthy and elastic. A good source of vitamin C is citrus fruit.

Skin Tags

Skin tags are small, loose growths of skin that appear under your arms or boobs. There's nothing you can do during pregnancy to get rid of these, at least not that I am aware of. However, after pregnancy, they often disappear. If they don't, you can have them removed.

Itchy Belly

As your baby bump gets bigger, your skin stretches and tightens. This can cause dryness and itching.

Tip: Keep the area moisturised with natural oils. I found that refrigerated almond oil helped a lot, so pop some in the fridge and have it on hand for itchy times.

You can also use calamine lotion if it's really itchy but the oil was enough for me. Some people swear by oatmeal baths but I'm not sure how effective these are as I didn't try them.

If you experience severe itching late in your pregnancy, possibly accompanied by nausea, vomiting, a loss of appetite, fatigue and jaundice, you should contact your doctor. You might have cholestasis, a treatable liver problem.

Linea Nigra

Around the fifth month of pregnancy, a dark line appears on your tummy. For me, it seemed to come out of nowhere, but I've been told by others that it appears gradually. Mine looked as though a tattoo artist had started to paint a tree and forgot the leaves and branches. It was that prominent. What might surprise you is that, pregnant or not, everyone has the line, but most people probably never notice it pre pregnancy because it's light-coloured. During pregnancy, the line darkens due to those oh-so-reliable hormones. There's not a whole pile you can do to prevent the *linea nigra* during pregnancy, other than taming it by staying out of direct sunlight. Direct sunlight will make it worse. Thankfully, the line should fade naturally with time, although there are no guarantees.

Tip: Apply a mixture of cider vinegar and lemon juice to the line. With a cotton bud, dab the mixture onto the line three times daily. I did this myself and my line disappeared within a few months. Make sure not to go on either side of it as the mixture lightens skin. The last thing you want is a white line running down your tummy!

Stretch Marks

Stretch marks rank high on the most dreaded aspects of pregnancy list so I have devoted the next chapter to discussing them in detail. They can not only impact tummy appearance, they can really affect confidence, as so many women will tell you. Our aim is to avoid getting them in the first place!

There is a lot of information out there about the prevention and treatment of stretch marks, but most of it is rubbish and confusing, in my opinion. There are many companies claiming to offer solutions, but they cannot back up their claims with real-life results. These products might smell nice and work in theory but unless I've seen it really work on other women or I've used it myself and got results, I don't buy it.

I wanted to make sure I didn't get stretch marks so, after a lot of research, I put together my own method and my own product. And I haven't a single stretch mark.

4
Stretch Marks

Technically, stretch marks are called *stria* or *striae*, and *striae gravidarum* during pregnancy. Pregnant women are the most common victims of the ghastly things, but puberty and bodybuilding can cause them too. They commonly pop up on the tummy, under-arms, inner thighs, boobs, biceps and bum. They are usually red and purple to begin with, but generally fade down to a silver colour, as though that's any con-solation.

Causes of Stretch Marks

We all know that stretch marks are caused by over-stretching, but there's an important aspect of their for-mation that is rarely taken into account and needs to be if we are to prevent them. It's not just the stretch-ing process of the skin that is responsible for stretch marks. Now take a deep breath before you read the next couple of sentences. Glucocorticoid hormones in the body can prevent fibroblasts (cells in connective tissue that produce collagen and other fibres) in the skin from forming collagen. This means that the skin is less elastic. As a result, it is not as capable of handling all the stretching and the dermis and epidermis layers begin to tear. Now there's a mouthful for you! In not-so-sciencey language, hormones cause your skin to lose elasticity so it finds it hard to accommodate the stretching. Let's take a look at this graphically.

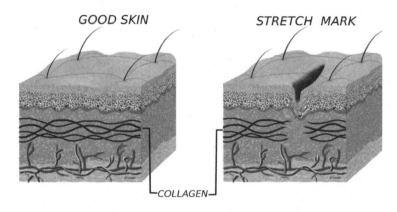

The important part to note is that stretch marks occur in the dermis when the skin is overstretched over a short period of time, such as when you're pregnant. The rapid stretching causes the dermis to tear. The biological intelligence behind this is to relieve pressure, a genius system – if only it weren't so ugly. As the dermis tissue starts to repair itself, the smooth appearance of normal skin is lost, hence the raised look of stretch marks. This is exactly what happens when any part of the body gets cut for any reason. Ultimately, stretch marks are scars, so they should be treated in the same way.

If we are to prevent stretch marks, we must prevent the dermis from ripping in the first place. If you have already got stretch marks we must work on smoothing out your skin and encouraging new skin growth, which is doable, but our primary aim here is to prevent them.

You could liken skin to chewing gum. When gum is chewed it becomes elastic. As a result, it stretches easily and to rip it would actually be quite difficult. If a piece of gum has not yet gone through that process of becoming more elastic, all you have to do is give it a gentle tug and it will come apart, leaving a jagged edge. We need to make sure that our skin, like our chewing gum, goes through a process of becoming more elastic, so it won't tear.

So how can we make your skin more *stretchable*? If I were to ask you to make gum more stretchable, what would you tell me to do? Add saliva? Yes! And what is saliva? Water! Wouldn't you agree that it's very difficult to break something when it's wet? It is essential then that you hydrate your skin and eliminate any dryness from the inside out and the outside in.

Hydration

When hydrating your skin it is essential that you avoid anything that might dry it out. There's no point to getting your skin all lovely and hydrated and then undoing our good work two seconds later. Here are some dos and don'ts.

Don'ts

- Caffeine: You should avoid caffeine throughout pregnancy anyway as doing so is much better for your baby, but another reason for avoiding it is because it dries your skin. Caffeine lurks in coffee, tea, soda and energy drinks, so you may be downing more of it than you think. It also acts a diuretic. In other words, it makes you pee more. And, being pregnant, you're probably doing more than enough of that already!

- Long periods of sun exposure: The sun robs your skin of moisture. It's not rocket science. If it rains and the sun comes out for ten minutes, what happens to the ground? It dries!

- Processed or salty foods such as processed or salted meats, fried foods, white breads and sugary snacks

- Soap: It robs your skin of moisture like you wouldn't believe. Instead of soap bars use a mild, fragrance-free wash.

- Scrubbing: Friction strips the skin so be gentle when washing.

- Harsh exfoliation: Exfoliation is excellent for getting rid of dead skin and promoting new growth, but it should be done gently, properly and with natural exfoliators.

- Lost shower moisture: Showering bathes your skin in moisture, which is perfect. Scrubbing yourself dry with a towel right afterward strips that moisture away. The surface of your skin absorbs some of the water, which will be lost if you don't seal it in. Pat yourself dry after a shower, do not scrub.

- Hot showers: A piping-hot shower can feel great when everything around you is freezing, but it strips your skin of its natural oils. Have warm, not hot, showers.

- Dry air: Indoor heating strips moisture from the air and your skin suffers as a result. Ease off the thermostat!

- Lotions: They might smell lovely and have pretty packaging but they will eventually make you look shabby. Stick to natural oils, such as olive oil, sweet almond oil, canola oil, castor oil, safflower oil, sesame seed oil or wheat germ oil. Or use a natural gel such as pure aloe vera gel. Add something to make it smell nice, if you like. Sandalwood, lavender oil and orange oil smell good and they are used to add fragrance to a lot of shop-bought lotions.

The bottom line is that you should protect your skin from water-robbing circumstances and, most importantly, hydrate it with water and moisture-rich compounds. So what can we do to hydrate your skin?

Dos

- Drink water: You've been told a thousand times to drink eight glasses of water a day, right? Big whoop, it's not breaking news but, as I said earlier, you need to drink more water when you're pregnant. The interesting bit here is that I recommend drinking a specific type of water, the water I drank throughout my pregnancy, the water I still drink. The water I recommend, based on my own experience and the documented research available, is alkaline water. It is shown to be perfect during pregnancy and I will explain why I drink it.

    - The pH of something can range from one to fourteen, one being totally acidic and fourteen being totally alkaline. Our body should have a pH balance of about 7.35. In reality, the majority of people in Western societies have a very acidic pHs. Not good! Think about it for a moment, if I was to take your hand and dip it in a bucket of acid what would happen? It would burn, right? The stomach has a pH of about 2. What happens to food when it hits the stomach? It breaks down into liquid, right? Acid rots and burns, simple as that. Here's the scary bit: tap water, bottled water and dispenser water are all acidic. If you test their acid levels they will show pH levels of about 3.5, only 1.5 away from your stomach's pH! You can test this yourself using litmus paper, reagent drops or a digital meter, which can be got from pharmacists. Reagent drops are the most accurate way of measuring pH, although the others are fairly good guides. The drops are simple to use with great, visual results that are easily understood. They work simply by changing colour due to reaction with alkalinity or acidity. The main ingredient in reagent drops is ethylene glycol, a highly reactive solution that catalyzes with any shift in pH and causes the dyes in reagent drops to shift colour accordingly. By simply comparing these colours to a pH chart, you can easily obtain a close approximation of a clear liquid's pH value.

○ Considering the pH of water, bottled water and dispenser water, it means that the majority of people are pouring acid into their systems every couple of hours and they don't even know it. Is it any wonder that illness and skin conditions are so prevalent in Western society? In the simplest of terms, acid causes disease and strips the skin. So girlie, to hydrate your skin and help your body I recommend that you drink alkalized water (something with a pH of 9 to 9.5 is perfect). You can buy an alkalizing filter to attach to your tap and, of course, you can check with your doctor to make sure you feel comfortable with the water you drink.

- Eat hydrating foods:

  ○ Omega-3 fatty acids: Your skin has a natural barrier to help it retain moisture, and that barrier contains omega-3 fatty acids. Omega-3 fatty acids are traditionally known as 'brain food', but they are also hugely beneficial to your skin, moisturising it from deep inside. These 'good fats' keep your skin moist, prevent sagging and collagen breakdown, and fight against nasty free radicals. They will also help your baby's development, so make sure to get lots of omega-3s during pregnancy. Signs that you have a deficiency would be if you suffer from premature wrinkles, dry skin, dandruff or cracked skin. Having said that, whether you are deficient or not, get loads of omega-3s. This will help your skin to perform the way you want it to, helping to prevent stretch marks and the saggy pouch. Good sources of omega-3s are oily fish, flax seeds and walnut oil. However, possibly the best source, the source I used right through my pregnancy is chia seed. Many people have never even heard of chia seed but it is fantastic. Used by the Aztecs, it is said to have more than five hundred percent more omega-3 than wild salmon and the tiny seeds are tasteless so they can be sprinkled on anything really. You wouldn't even know you were eating them. I put mine in my daily beauty smoothie, the recipe for which you will find later in this book.

o Lutein: Taking just ten milligrams of lutein, the green pigment in plants, every day has been shown to boost skin hydration by sixty percent, skin elasticity by twenty percent and the levels of skin lipids by fifty percent. You can get it in green vegetables and fruits, such as cabbage, lettuce, broccoli, endives, asparagus, spinach, nettles, kiwi fruit, green apples, beans, peas, parsley and pepper grass.

- Vitamin E: Don't bother with expensive vitamin E-enriched creams. Chances are there is only a tiny blob of it in anything claiming to be a vitamin E cream. Instead, get vitamin E capsules or concentrated vitamin E oil from the health store. Massage it into your skin using small circular movements, preferably after a shower, when your pores are open.

- Kelp: It has one of the highest levels of minerals from any one source and is an excellent moisturiser. During my pregnancy, I took kelp supplements, but the ideal thing would be to get it in its natural form.

- Stevia: A natural, calorie-free sugar substitute, the stevia plant has very good hydrating effects. Stevia contains lots of antioxidants and helps to smooth out wrinkles. It's a beauty plant!

- Water-rich fruits and vegetables: Fruits and vegetables are good for you in so many ways but, when it comes to hydrating the skin, certain ones are particularly good. I hate celery. To me, celery tastes like rotten dandelions, not that I have ever tried rotten dandelions, but you get what I mean. Most people like it though and I hope you're one of them, as it's a superfood for hydrating your skin. In fact, it's ninety-six percent water and provides sodium, potassium, magnesium, calcium, phosphorus, iron and zinc.

○ Watermelon I could eat all day! When I was pregnant I ate loads of it. It is ninety-five per-cent water, is rich in vitamin C and tastes scrumptious. Bell peppers can be added to lots of things and are ninety-two percent water. They are also rich in vitamin C.

○ You can put cucumber slices on your eyes during a facial, but then put the rest of it in your mouth. It is about ninety-five percent water and it provides calcium, magnesium, sodium and potassium.

○ Strawberries are delicious eaten whole but also gorgeous in smoothies! They are ninety-two percent water and are rich in potassium.

Tissue Repair and Promoting New Skin Growth

- Vitamin B5: If you have stretch marks or if you haven't, it is important to take vitamin B5 to boost skin function and tissue repair. Avocados, yoghurt, mushrooms, sun-dried tomatoes and corn are good sources of vitamin B5. B vitamins, in general, are important to include in your diet; they can even influence your mood.

- Selenium: This mineral boosts the activity of antioxidants and helps to maintain the skin's elasticity. You can get the recommended daily amount by eating just four or five Brazil nuts!

- Exfoliation: Taking off dead skin cells allows for the growth of new ones. This is particularly important if you already have stretch marks. There are two steps you should take. First, 'dry brush' every day. There's no need to get an expensive body brush, a baby brush is just as effective. Gently brush your skin in upwards strokes, toward your heart and out to your armpits. This increases blood flow and helps the lymphatic system. Do not scrub. The aim is to lift only the top layer of cells, so gentle strokes are perfect. Second, use an exfoliating moisturiser. Instead of shop-bought junk, make a natural moisturising, exfoliating scrub using a combination of olive oil and sugar and use it ever other day. Combine a half a cup of sugar with two tablespoons of olive oil. Add lavender oil for a natural fragrance and coriander or cypress oil to improve circulation and lymphatic detox. Gently rub it all over your tummy, boobs, thighs, hips and bum using small circular movements. Wash it off gently.

Stretch-Mark Products

When I was researching stretch marks I looked at hundreds of products, most claiming to be miracle products, many of which had hefty price tags. However, when I looked behind the claims, the results disappointed me. The ingredients simply didn't coincide with how stretch marks form or with how skin behaves. So I looked at what natural products women were using to tackle stretch marks, things from all over the globe and across many different cultures. To my delight, women seemed to be having more success with natural ingredients and products. However, full prevention didn't seem evident anywhere when it came to big babies, bad genes, etc. Sure, some women didn't get stretch marks, but their babies were average-sized or stretch marks were not a common thing in their families. I knew I was having a whopper and genes weren't on my side.

With no alternative that I was willing to chance, I decided to make my own product, based on what I had seen to be somewhat effective in nature and using my knowledge of skin biology and chemistry. I would create a new, easily absorbed formula and put it to the test. I used it every day, twice a day, and took photos before, during and after my pregnancy. As you can see, the results speak for themselves. The first photo was taken when I was two-months pregnant, the second was taken in the hospital on the day of delivery, the third was taken two months post preg-nancy and the fourth was taken one year post preg-nancy. The photos were taken using my phone, which is why they don't look that professional, but at least they allow you to see my skin in its raw form. As you can see, not a stretch mark in sight.

Donna Kennedy

Two Months Pregnant

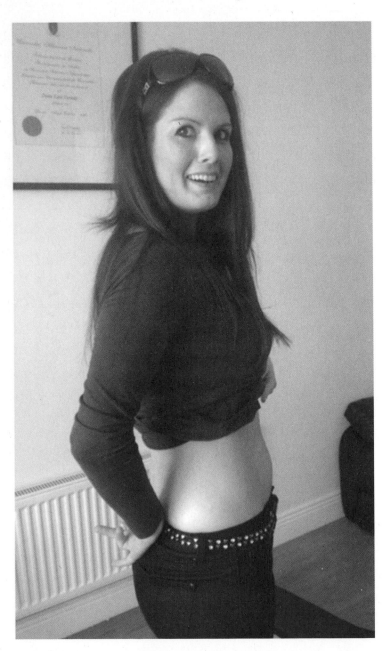

Full Term

I took this photo during the early stages of labour. You can't get more full term than that!

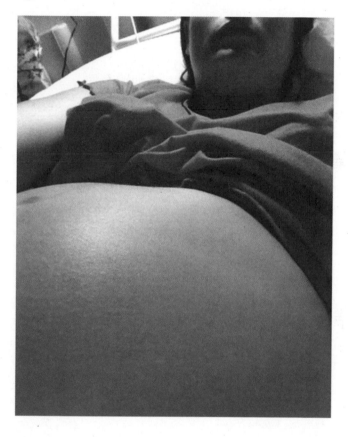

Two Months Post Pregnancy

You can see that at this stage I still had a *linea nigra*, although it had started to lighten in colour. However, I had no stretch marks whatsoever and I was in very good shape, having followed the *Born to Be Beautiful* pregnancy plan. Please note that I took this photo myself so, unfortunately you can't see my face. I hadn't planned on it being in a book! However, in the next photo I made sure to wear the same clothes and got someone else to take the photo so you know for sure it is me!

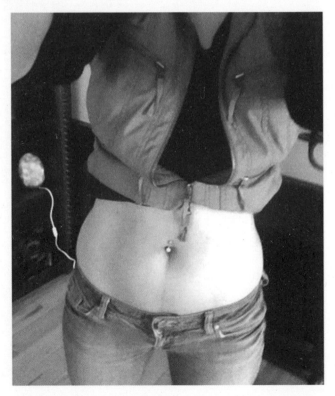

One Year Post Pregnancy with My Gorgeous Baby Boy, Ashton!

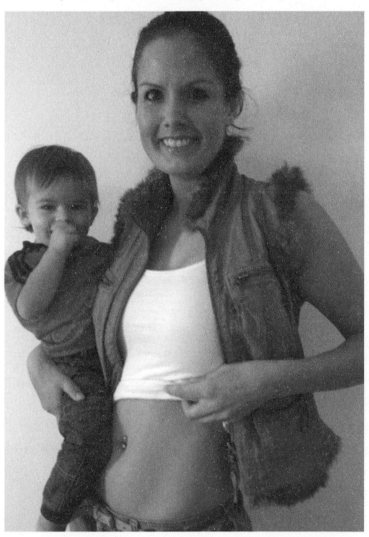

5
Eat!

As you can see from the first photo of me in Chapter 4, I had a lovely tummy when I was two months pregnant. Fast forward to my delivery date (as seen in the second photo) and I had a toad tummy, albeit a smooth, mark-free one. I felt really unattractive at that point, although I did feel good knowing I had prevented stretch marks and not gained much unwanted weight.

When I found out I was pregnant, which was at just three weeks, I had three aims. One was to prevent stretch marks, the second was to maintain my pre-pregnancy toned physique, and the third was to maintain my feeling of emotional well-being. I could tick off number one – I had prevented stretch marks – and I am delighted to say that using the *Born to Be Beautiful* pregnancy plan allowed me to maintain my figure and to feel amazing, better than I had ever felt. And it will allow you to do the same.

Whether you are thinking about getting pregnant, are currently pregnant or have already given birth, the

Born to Be Beautiful pregnancy plan applies. This plan does not involve starving, calorie counting or strict regimes. It is straightforward and it is designed to fit in with your lifestyle as a mother.

Become Friends with Your Body

It's important that you enjoy your life and to do that you need to respect your body. If you want amazing results long-term you must work with your body, not against it. The easiest way to do that is to become friends with your body. Get to know it, how it works, how it burns fat, how it tones itself, what it wants and what it loves. Then treat it well by working the *Born to Be Beautiful* pregnancy plan. It will perform brilliantly for you. Simply by eating specific foods and doing specific movements you will look and feel amazing in no time at all.

Eat!

It is a myth that the less you eat the more weight you will lose. The reality of it is that your body does not like it when you don't eat enough food and it will fight you all the way to make sure you feed it. This is why diets don't work. Starving will cause you to lose weight temporarily, no doubt, but as soon as you start eating properly again you will pile the weight back on, and maybe even more weight than you had in the first place. You see, your body has an inbuilt defence mechanism. It knows to do everything it can to keep you alive and safe, keep you warm and give you enough energy to live. If you oppose it, it will fight back.

In years gone by, when food wasn't as easily accessible as it is now, this was essential to survival. We were given the ability to find food and we were even given a reserve tank, in the event we couldn't find food for a while. Your body's reserve is fat. If you starve your body and try to fight the reserve, what do you think your body will do? Of course, like a child with its favourite toy, it will hold on tighter if you try to take it away. This is why people who yo-yo diet are never slim, despite great effort. They fight their body's natural metabolisms by dieting. As soon as their brain recognises that there's a diet in place, it shoots a rapid lock-down message to their body: *Hold on to your reserve for dear life*! A little while later, when the diet is eventually abandoned and the person starts to eat again, instead of their body working with them, it fights them and refuses to play ball. It won't let go of the fat, in case any kind of starvation is attempted again, the same as a child won't give you the toy in case you take it away again.

In light of this, it is much more useful (and nicer!) to become friends with your body and respect it. The key to doing this is learning what your body responds to best. When it comes to weight loss, your body wants and needs two things: a reserve of *good* fat and lean muscle.

Fat

Fat is *not* your enemy. Your body needs it. All your body wants is for you to give it the right amount of the right types of fats. Without fat, vitamins A, D, E and K can't be absorbed properly and they are so important to having a healthy, gorgeous body. The right kind of fats can actually help you to lose unwanted fat! Yes, you read it right – fat can help you *lose* unwanted fat. For the purposes of this book, we'll call the right kinds of fats 'good fats'.

Omega-3, omega-6 and omega-9 fatty acids, as well as monounsaturated fats, are the fats your body loves, the ones that it uses best. They have been shown to be very beneficial for health and weight loss, and you'll be delighted to know that a diet rich in monounsaturated fats prevents the accumulation of abdominal fat – great news for us mothers. Avoid saturated fats found in meat, lard, cream and whole dairy, and focus on getting good fats into your diet. Good fats are found in high-oleic sunflower oil, safflower oil, olive oil and canola oil, as well as in olives, avocadoes, granola, hazelnuts, almonds, peanuts, corn, sesame, rice bran, soybeans, mixed seeds, chia seed and oily fish.

Getting enough unsaturated fat in your diet can also help to curb hunger in two ways. First, an unsaturated fatty acid called oleic acid stimulates oleoylethanolamide (OEA) production. Increasing your OEA levels has been shown to reduce appetite, promote weight loss and lower cholesterol. High levels of oleic acid can be found in olive oil, rapeseed oil, hazelnuts (oil-roasted and salted), peanut oil and macadamia nuts (roasted and salted). Second, omega-3 fatty acids cause your body to increase the amount of the hormone leptin in your system. Leptin is known for suppressing hunger. A good way to get omega fatty acids if you don't like oil, which I'm not a lover of, is to put chia seed into a smoothie and down it with delight.

Muscle – The 'Bad Fat' Buster!

In order to help your body burn unnecessary fat it is essential that you create a fat-burning tool. That tool is muscle. No need to worry, I have no intention of turning you into the Hulk. All we want to do is create enough muscle in your body so your metabolism speeds up and you automatically burn any unnecessary fat, staying feminine and toned in the process.

Muscle, by definition, is the soft tissue of animals. It is made up of cells that contain protein filaments that slide past one another to produce a contraction, so we can move. If we are to create more muscle what do you think you might need? Of course, you need protein. It is the only way you will create a decent fat-burning tool so, needless to say, it is an important part of the *Born to Be Beautiful* pregnancy plan.

Protein

High-protein foods need more energy from the body to process, thus the fat-burning properties. To work, the *Born to Be Beautiful* pregnancy plan most effectively you need to focus on eating more protein but, more importantly, you need to focus on eating quality protein. Your body actually has protein preferences: it will accept and use certain proteins faster than others and some proteins can't easily be used by the body at all. Since we want to fast-track everything, we need you to eat lots of quality protein. At least thirty percent of your diet should be protein-based.

To determine how useful protein is for your body, we need to look at the building blocks which make up protein, amino acids. There are twenty main amino acids in protein, nine of which your body cannot make on its own. They are essential and you have to get them from your diet. Not only that, they must come in the right ratios to be used effectively. I'm not expecting you to figure out all the science. All I want you to do is eat the right types of protein.

In my opinion, the best proteins to eat are egg whites (well-cooked) and quinoa (pronounced 'keen-wah'), as they are easily used by the body. Quinoa can be bought in most health stores. Not only is it a complete protein, containing eight amino acids (including lysine), it's packed full of dietary fibre, phosphorus, magnesium, vitamin E, potassium and iron. It's also gluten-free and easy to digest. It looks a bit like couscous and is as versatile as rice, so make sure to stock your cupboard with it. Cooked, it lasts for a few days in the fridge, or up to one month in the freezer.

Eat Often

The *Born to Be Beautiful* pregnancy plan involves eating several meals a day. The key is eating small amounts of the right foods often so your body keeps your metabolism running nicely, like a car ticks over properly when it has the right amount of the correct fuel in it.

Sugar

Sugar influences hunger and metabolism so, needless to say, your body does not want you to eliminate sugar but it does want you to give it the best type. You can do this easily by referring to a food's glycaemic index (GI), a figure representing the speed and extent to which it releases sugar into the bloodstream. Just look at the list I have included in this book or at GI lists on good nutritional websites. In a nutshell, the higher a food's GI, the less satisfied your body feels and the more you want to eat. To combat hunger and metabolism issues, simply opt for low-GI foods. This means limiting *refined* sugars, i.e. foods containing white flour, such as breads, cakes, regular pastas and breakfast cereals, as well as foods with white sugar, such as candy and chocolate. You must eat carbohydrates as they are good for energy, but your body responds better to those it can use for energy throughout the day, not just for a few minutes. When you eat starchy refined carbs your body finds it difficult to digest them and, as a result, your blood sugar yo-yos so you get hungry quickly and often. When your body eats good carbs, it releases a hormone called 'glucagon-like peptide 1' into your gut to give you a feeling of fullness. When you feel full you have no desire to overeat. Have a look at this list and you can begin to make some food adjustments straight away.

Glycaemic Index (GI) Examples

Breakfast Cereals

Low GI	Medium GI	High GI
All-Bran	Nutrigrain	Cornflakes
Oat bran	Shredded wheat	Sultana Bran
Rolled oats	Special K (USA)	Branflakes
Special K (UK/Aus)	Instant porridge	Rice Krispies
Natural muesli		
Porridge		

Breads

Low GI	Medium GI	High GI
Whole wheat	Croissant	White
Sourdough rye	Hamburger bun	Bagel
Sourdough wheat	White pita	French baguette
Heavy mixed grain		
Soya and linseed		
Wholegrain		
Pumpernickle		

Staples

Low GI	Medium GI	High GI
New potatoes	Basmati rice	Instant white rice
Tortellini (cheese)	Couscous	Glutinous rice
Egg fettuccini	Cornmeal	Short-grain white rice
Brown rice	Taco shells	Tapioca
Buckwheat	Gnocchi	Mashed potatoes
Long-grain white rice	Canned potatoes	French fries
Wheat tortillas	Chinese rice	
Wheat pasta	Baked potatoes	

Snacks

Low GI	Medium GI	High GI
Walnuts	Blueberry muffins	Pretzels
Peanuts	Digestives	Water crackers
Nuts and raisins	Honey	Rice cakes
Hummus	Ryvita	Scones
Oatmeal crackers		
Cashew nuts		

Vegetables

Low GI	Medium GI	High GI
Frozen green peas	Beetroot	Pumpkin
Frozen sweet corn	Fresh corn	Parsnips
Carrots		
Eggplant/aubergine		
Broccoli		
Cauliflower		
Cabbage		

Fruits

Low GI	Medium GI	High GI
Cherries	Mango	Dates
Plums	Sultanas	Watermelons
Grapefruit	Bananas	
Peaches	Raisins	
Apples	Papaya	
Pears	Figs	
Grapes	Pineapple	
Kiwi Fruit		

Dairy

Low GI	Medium GI	High GI
Whole milk	Ice cream	Sweetened yoghurt
Skimmed milk		
Chocolate milk		
Artificially sweetened Yoghurt		
Custard		
Soy milk		

Legumes (Beans)

All beans and peas are low GI apart from canned kidney beans, which are medium GI.

'Satiety Foods': Foods That Fill You Up

Throughout my pregnancy, and indeed before and after it, I ate what are known as 'satiety foods'. These are foods that fill you up fast and speed up your metabolism, while satisfying every nutritional desire your body has. By eating satiety foods, it's much easier to stay at a healthy weight. No cravings and a full tummy – all part of the plan! Here is an A-Z list of some 'fill-me-up' foods that you can add to your meals. You will find a vast list online, but this list will get you started.

Tip: Chew your food properly. The human brain takes approximately twenty minutes to register a feeling of fullness. Chewing slows down eating, which encourages the brain to release the enzymes that register the full feeling. It also makes food easier to digest.

A

Apples: An apple a day can keep weight gain at bay. Handy on the go or as a snack, apples are great for filling the gap between meals. In one study, people who ate an apple before a pasta meal ate fewer calories overall than those who had a different snack. Plus, the antioxidants in apples can help prevent metabolic syndrome, a condition marked by excess tummy fat. You can eat an apple on its own or, for a pie-like treat, chop it up, sprinkle it with half a teaspoon of allspice and half a teaspoon of cinnamon, and pop it in the microwave for a minute and a half.

Apple-cider vinegar: Just one and a half tablespoons of apple cider vinegar can make you eat two hundred fewer calories at your next meal. The likely reason for this is that vinegar tends to blunt blood insulin levels that trigger hunger. Vinegar or lemon juice with high-carb foods lowers any sudden increase in blood sugar. So all round a good'n!

B

Beans: Full of protein and fibre, beans are a super-food for filling you up. There are lots of varieties, so they can be used in many different ways: hot on baked potatoes and in stews, or cold in salads. I love a mix of kidney beans and butter beans served with mint vinaigrette.

Bananas: Not only are bananas sweet and fairly inexpensive, they provide energy and nutrition without fat. They also contain resistant starch, a great boon for weight loss (and your overall health). Resistant starch doesn't get absorbed into the bloodstream in the small intestine like other foods. Instead, as it passes through the system, it creates a chain reaction, shrinking fat cells, preserving muscle, stoking your metabolism and making you feel fuller for longer. A slightly green, medium-size banana will fill you up between meals and boost your metabolism with its twelve and a half grams of resistant starch. A ripe banana still ranks high on the list of foods containing resistant starch, with almost five grams.

Balsamic Vinegar: Beautiful drizzled on a salad or added to a hot dish, balsamic vinegar boosts production of digestion enzymes, improving your metabolism and giving you a full feeling.

C

Cayenne pepper: According to recent research published in the journal *Physiology & Behaviour*, just half a teaspoon of cayenne pepper can boost your metabolism and cause your body to burn an extra ten calories on its own.

Not to mention that, for those who don't regularly eat spicy meals, adding cayenne pepper can cut an average of sixty calories from a meal. Do that two meals a day for a month and you'll lose four pounds without even trying!

Chilli: A compound in chilli called capsaicin has a thermogenic effect, meaning it causes the body to burn extra calories for twenty minutes after you eat them.

Cinnamon: Next time you have cereal, oatmeal or fruit, sprinkle some cinnamon on it. Cinnamon helps lower your blood sugar levels, which – you guessed it – helps to control your appetite!

D

Dips: Noshing on vegetables is a classic weight-management strategy, but you'll feel full longer if you allow yourself a little savoury dip to go along with those carrot and zucchini sticks. The flavour and the fat will keep you feeling full longer and can help your body absorb nutrients like beta-carotene more effectively. Try a little salad dressing, or whip up a batch of delicious hummus.

Dark chocolate: I'm not an advocate of chocolate to be honest, but if you feel you'd like some, go for dark chocolate. The bittersweet taste can help suppress your appetite. Chocolate is high in calories and refined sugars, so eat it in small portions. Not all chocolate is an appetite suppressant, only dark chocolate.

E

Egg-white omelettes: Fry egg whites in a little olive oil (to get your omegas) and flavour with mushrooms and red onions or tomato and red onions.

F

Flax seeds: A great plant source of omega-3 fatty acids, flax seeds are also very high in protein and fibre, making them excellent for appetite control. Sprinkle ground flax seeds over oatmeal, salads or yogurt, or add them to smoothies to help stabilise your blood sugar and turn off the hunger hormones.

G

Green vegetables: Vegetables like cabbage or broccoli are high in fibre and require extra time and energy in the digestion process. You feel full longer and, as a bonus, you will burn extra calories in digestion.

Ginger: A stimulant that energises the body and kickstarts digestion, ginger root works especially well in Indian dishes. Gingerbread men don't count!

Green tea: An appetite suppressant that has fat-burning potential, green tea has thermogenic effects that burn calories and can help your body burn fat.

H

Hoodia: A succulent plant native to Africa, interest in hoodia's use for appetite control and weight loss was piqued by reports of hunters using it to reduce hunger during long hunts. You can get it in African stores and some health stores. Do not take this plant during your pregnancy. It is intended for after pregnancy.

I

Ice pops: Make natural ice pops using smoothie mix or fresh, homemade juice. They are delicious and great to have as a grab-and-go treat.

J

Juice: Every day I drink a pint of fresh juice. I make it myself, juicing four apples, a carrot, half a cucumber and a quarter of a fresh lime. I know it sounds gross but all I can say is try it before you knock it. I know you'll love it and, after you taste it, you'll want it to be part of your food plan. Adding some green vegetables is great too, and you won't really taste them. As I said, try it before you knock it!

K

Kiwi fruit: An easy grab-and-go snack food. Full of fibre, it's a super alternative to junk food.

L

Lean protein: I am a vegetarian so my protein comes from these sources: eggs, whey, cheese and nuts. If you are not a vegetarian, focus on lean proteins such as fish and chicken. Combine protein with a low-GI carb for maximum effect, as it is used more easily by the body this way.

Lentils: Bona fide tummy flatteners, lentils help to prevent insulin spikes that cause your body to create excess fat, especially in the abdominal area. There are many varieties of lentils so play around with them by adding spices and sauces.

M

Melons: High in water and low in calories, melons are a perfect and tasty solution to any sweet craving. They have naturally occurring sugars, which can help satisfy a sweet tooth and allow you to resist eating high-calorie, rubbish food.

N

Nuts: They don't just contain healthy fats – they are also good sources of appetite-killing fibre, which digests slowly so it stays in your stomach much longer than other carbohydrates. A quarter cup of almonds, for example, contains four grams of fibre. Nuts are also a good source of protein.

O

Oatmeal: While high in carbs, the type of carbs in oatmeal is slow-digesting and keeps you feeling full for hours after breakfast. Why? They suppress the hunger hormone ghrelin. In fact, oatmeal is pretty low on the glycaemic index – just be sure to use steel-cut oats to get the most benefit.

P

Pine nuts: Pine nuts contain more protein than any other type of nut or seed, and they have appetite-suppressing pinolenic acid, which naturally reduces hunger.

Potatoes: Potatoes contain a special type of starch that resists digestive enzymes, making them stay in your body longer, causing you not to get hungry for long periods of time. However, don't eat processed potatoes like French fries or potato chips, which are loaded with unhealthy fats, salts, sugars and additives. Instead, eat baked potatoes served with beans, tuna and sweet corn, low-fat coleslaw or salad. Boiled baby potatoes are lovely with Mojo sauce, a spicy Canarian blend of chilli, spices, olive oil and cider vinegar. Seriously delicious!

Popcorn: With only about fifty-five calories per cup, popcorn takes up a lot of space in the stomach, helping to create feelings of fullness.

Q

Quinoa: With a stellar nutrient combo, quinoa can keep you satisfied for hours. Serve it instead of rice with stir-fries, lentils and curries. It's a much better alternative!

R

Rye bread: Proven to increase satiety, rye bread suppresses your hunger and the desire to snack on foods throughout the day. So, if you start the day with rye bread for breakfast, your appetite will be reduced before lunch and into the afternoon.

S

Soup: If you have soup before a meal, you're going to eat less, simple as that. The good thing is that there are many flavours of soup to choose from. Make sure to cook your soup yourself, though, and throw in lots of green veg. Greens will make the soup alkaline, give you lots of nutrients and fill you up fast. One important thing to note is that cream is not a good ingredient in soup. It contains bad fats that will not do you any favours, so leave it out. If you put in enough veg and season it well you won't need it anyway.

Tip: Freeze portions of soup so you have it on hand if you feel peckish.

Smoothies: Every day during pregnancy I had a pint of 'beauty smoothie' (I still do). It's my own recipe and the reason I call it 'beauty smoothie' is because it has everything to give you the nutrients necessary to make you beautiful. It's full of antioxidants, vitamins, minerals, absorbable calcium, omega-3 fatty acids, alkaline compounds and protein – a total superfood and really filling! The recipe can be found in the appendix at the back of this book.

Tip: Make the smoothie thick, like a sorbet. It feels like a meal in itself. Put some of the mixture in ice-pop moulds and freeze them for grab-and-go treats.

Spirulina: A superfood that contains over a hundred nutrients, spirulina can be bought in powder form or in capsules in most health stores. I always put it in my smoothies. Since it is a microalga, it contains high levels of minerals that are frequently lacking in modern diets, such as magnesium. It is known to reduce cravings for sweets and carbohydrates. Not only that, it is a great source of protein, contains lots of B vitamins and is very alkaline. Make sure you get a high-quality brand that clearly indicates that the spirulina has been cultivated in non-toxic waters. This is important, as some low-quality brands cultivate it in unclean conditions, which can be harmful to you.

T

Tofu: As a rich, plant-based protein source, tofu isn't just for vegetarians! It is high in an isoflavone called genistein, which has been shown to suppress appetite and lower food intake. For an easy way to introduce tofu to your diet, try adding it to your next healthy stir fry. On its own, tofu is spongy, but it can be really nice when it is cooked in a sauce – especially a Thai sauce.

U

Umeboshi: Can't control your sweet tooth? In Eastern medicine, foods are regarded as having certain properties and a craving for one kind of food (a sweet food, for example) can best be treated by eating its opposite (a bitter food). Umeboshi, which are basically pickled plums, are the ultimate in 'contractive' foods and are great for sugar cravings. You can get them in Asian stores. If you find yourself with a craving for sugar, try dipping a spoon into a jar of umeboshi paste and licking it off. The sourness will give you a jolt.

V

Vegetable kebabs: There are lots of veg kebab variations. Add cheese cubes, fruit, or whatever takes your fancy. But a really nice kebab can be made using bell peppers, eggplants, button mushrooms and yellow onions, marinated in a mixture of a quarter cup of balsamic vinegar, one tablespoon of Dijon mustard, one teaspoon of rosemary, one teaspoon of oregano, five cloves garlic (peeled and chopped), three tablespoons of olive oil, and some salt and cracked pepper. Delish!

W

Whey protein: Protein is known for suppressing appetite, but it seems that whey protein is especially good at it. Obviously you couldn't eat whey on its own, but put it in a smoothie and you wouldn't even know it was there. The recipe for my beauty smoothie is in the recipe section. Only use quality whey (with the advice of a nutritionist). There are some rubbish brands on the market.

X

Xanthones: Contained in a fruit called a mangosteen, xanthones are associated with increased fat metabolism. It's best to get the whole fruit, but that can be tricky. However, you can get mangosteen juice in health stores. Make sure it has not been blended with juices from other fruits and, to avoid sugar over-load, only drink a small glass of it.

Y

Yoghurt: Low-fat Greek yoghurt has a nice mixture of protein, fats and carbs, and is a good snack. Instead of buying fruit yoghurt though, which can be laden with sugar and additives, just add fresh berries, peaches, pears or pineapple to natural Greek yoghurt. Much nicer and really healthy!

Z

Zucchini (courgette): Foods that are high in fibre are good appetite suppressors. Zucchini is full of fibre. You can use zucchini by slicing it thinly into your hot dishes.

Important Note

Please consult your doctor to ensure that the foods mentioned here are appropriate for you and your baby. All appetite reducing foods or foods that help you lose weight should only be used *post* pregnancy and not until your doctor says it's okay.

6
The Born to Beautiful Movement Plan

During and after my pregnancy I did specific *movements* to maintain a healthy weight and stay toned. I say movements, not exercise, because I never broke a sweat. My lifestyle at the time didn't allow me to do any of the typical types of exercise advocated for pregnancy, such as swimming. So you can be confident that the things I did and that I am going to show you are very effective and safe.

I am the same as every other woman on the planet: my chances of putting on excess weight during pregnancy were as high as anyone else's and my chances of getting a saggy tummy were as high as anyone else's. When pregnant, we're all in the same boat. But as you can see from my photos, great results are possible if you do specific things.

I didn't use any expensive equipment. The *Born to Be Beautiful* pregnancy plan involves the floor, two small weights and an inexpensive stability ball. That's it! I started my plan early in my pregnancy and ideally you would do the same, but you can do this at any stage. Some of the movements are so easy that I did them as I brushed my teeth or fed my baby.

It's important to note, however, that no matter how simple a movement is, you should always consult with your doctor to make sure it's right for you, pregnant or not. You must do things at your own pace. I didn't do anything for a few weeks post pregnancy, as I under-went an episiotomy (ouch!) during my baby's delivery and I was too sore. The same would apply if you had a caesarean section. You'd need to be extra careful and possibly allow more time.

Building Strong Muscles During and After Pregnancy

During pregnancy, two muscle groups in particular are affected: those in the abdominal area and those in the pelvic area. The pectoral (chest) area can also be put under strain as a result of an increase in breast size during pregnancy. We will look at how all these mus-cles are affected and then I will show you how we can prevent damage and, if necessary, recondition.

Abdominal Changes

The organs in your tummy are covered by two large

muscle sheets, known as recti muscles. These cover the tummy and run from the rib cage down to the pubic bone. They meet in the middle of your tummy, in line with your belly button. Towards the end of pregnancy, these muscles can separate. Most women don't even know that the separation is happening, and if you have a premature baby it may not happen at all. If you have a caesarean it has to happen so the surgeon can access the baby. Your delivery stage or type will determine how much work you will need to do post pregnancy to achieve your desired physique, but you can do it!

Widening and Thinning

In conjunction with pregnancy hormones that soften connective tissue, widening and thinning of the midline tissue occurs in response to the force of the uterus pushing against the abdominal wall. Widening happens in all pregnancies but sometimes the muscles widen too much, i.e. more than two centimetres. Excessive separation of the midline is known as *diastasis recti* and it can happen any time in the last half of pregnancy. It occurs in about thirty percent of all pregnancies. It's most commonly seen after pregnancy, when the abdominal wall is lax and the thinner midline tissue no longer provides enough support for the torso and organs.

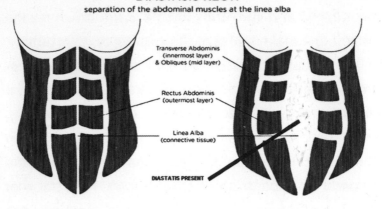

DIASTASIS RECTI
separation of the abdominal muscles at the linea alba

Signs of *Diastasis Recti*

- A gap of more than two and a half finger-widths when the *rectus abdominis* is fully contracted.

- The gap does not shrink as you contract your abdominal wall.

- You can see a small mound sticking out along the length of your midline.

Your doctor or midwife can confirm whether you have it or not, if you want to know.

Pelvic-Floor Muscles

The pelvic-floor area is formed by lots of soft tissues that fill the outlet of your pelvis. The most important of these is a strong sheet of muscles, slung like a hammock from the walls of the pelvis. The urethra, the vagina and the anal canal pass through these muscles.

They support the weight of the intestines, your uterus and your unborn baby. They can be blamed for all those trips to the bathroom during pregnancy. Pelvic-floor muscles soften and weaken to a degree during pregnancy, due to the hormone progesterone. It needs to happen so your baby can make its way into this world. The natural process of carrying your baby, along with its journey out, can further weaken the pelvic floor. This is why pelvic-floor exercises are important for all women throughout their lives, especially during and after pregnancy. Later on, I will show you the ones I did.

Things to Consider

I recommend that you start the *Born to Be Beautiful* pregnancy plan movements as soon as you learn you are pregnant, with your doctor's approval. Post pregnancy, it is recommended that you wait six weeks before you do any of the more complex movements shown here and before you exercise. How soon you start exercising is entirely up to you and your doctor. You must feel comfortable and you must allow your body to heal. Your safety and the safety of your baby are paramount. Following my episiotomy, I couldn't even sit comfortably for three weeks, never mind move about or exercise, so I just allowed myself to heal before doing anything. Thankfully, because I strengthened my muscles during pregnancy using *Born to Be Beautiful* movement and food plan, I had a strong core post pregnancy. My body immediately and naturally started to tone itself and, as the weeks progressed, I worked with it to get the results I wanted.

Things to Avoid

- Weighing yourself: Muscle is heavier than fat, so instead of measuring progress on the scales, measure it by how well your clothes fit. I never weigh myself. I just go by my clothes size. It's much more normal and you don't get the daily pressure of weight fluctuations, which you will naturally experience throughout your menstrual cycle.

- Backbends: You do not need to stretch yourself almost to the breaking point to get toned, and you definitely don't need to be bending backwards. Lying backwards over a large exercise ball, for example, may look cool but it is *not* a good exercise to do post pregnancy. It will put way too much strain on your muscles and could actually backfire, making your muscles go wonky.

- Abdominal crunches (oblique curls): Abdominal crunches can be damaging post pregnancy. They can actually worsen abdominal separation, and they can cause the pregnancy pouch. Instead, opt for the exercises outlined here. They are safer and much more effective.

- Lifting and carrying very heavy objects: Although obvious, I would like to remind you that lifting and carrying will put a strain on your muscles.

- Jumping out of bed: Help your tummy stay supported by getting out of bed slowly. When pregnant, with your torso and head aligned and in one piece, roll over onto your side. Then use your arms to push yourself up to a sitting position.

- Over-tilting your pelvis: When doing pelvic-floor movements, it is easy to over-tilt so be mindful and support your body when you do them.

Now it's time for action!

Born to Be Beautiful Movement Plan

To work the plan properly, there are a series of specific movements you need to do daily, in a specific sequence. I do not claim to be an expert. I am simply showing you exactly what I did to get my body back.

Pelvic-Floor Muscle Toning

Before pregnancy, I did what are known as Kegel exercises. These can help you prevent or control urinary incontinence and other pelvic-floor problems, and your midwife will recommend you do them anyway. Ideally, you would do these before and during pregnancy but don't worry about it if you start later.

First, find the right muscles. To identify your pelvic-floor muscles try to stop peeing midstream. If you succeed, you've got the right muscles. Once you've identified your pelvic-floor muscles, empty your bladder and lie on your back. Tighten your pelvic-floor muscles, hold the contraction for five seconds and then relax for five seconds.

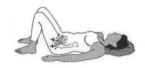

Do this four or five times in a row. Work up to keeping the muscles contracted for ten seconds at a time, relaxing for ten seconds between contractions. Repeat three times a day, and aim for ten repetitions per each set.

Tummy Toning

Most people would assume that to get a flat tummy we must do lots of tummy crunches. This couldn't be further from the truth. As I said, crunches aren't the way to get great looking abs at all, especially if you have *diastasis recti*. You'll just end up with a protruding midsection. To tighten your tummy, you need to work your entire core – meaning *all* the muscles in your abdomen. The series of movements that I am about to show you is super effective. Follow the steps laid out for you and do each movement in sequence three times per week.

Preparation
Have a clear image in your mind about what you want to look like. The more you focus on what you *do* want, the quicker your body will get you there. Bringing up my 'ideal self' gave me a clear target, a bit like how, when you're running a marathon you think about the finishing line, not every step you run. Keep the goal in mind, not just the process.

Doing the movements in front of a mirror – ideally

a big one – ensures that you are doing them correctly and allows you to measure your progress. Ignore your wobbly bits and focus on what you will look like when you get your desired body. Doing lots of fast movements will not get results and is not safe. Remember that muscles are like chewing gum. They should not be snapped, they should be stretched slowly and evenly.

A stability ball, sometimes known as a gym ball or a Swiss ball, is not expensive and can be purchased in most sports stores. It will give you super support for doing your movements and it will allow you to do movements that you wouldn't be able to do as effectively, or at all, on your own. It's important that you get one that's right for your height. This should be indicated on the box (they come deflated) but ask store staff if you are unsure which size to buy.

Movement 1: The Plank

A plank is an isometric core-strength exercise that involves maintaining a difficult position for an extended period of time. The most common plank is the traditional front plank, which is held in a push-up position with the body's weight borne on forearms, elbows, and toes, as shown in the following diagram. It is also called a front hold, a hover or an abdominal bridge. This is not a position I would recommend during pregnancy as it might be too strenuous for you and your baby.

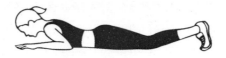

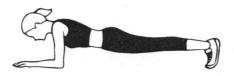

The purpose of the plank during and post pregnancy is to strengthen your core muscles, which are most challenged during pregnancy. By drawing your muscles upwards and inwards towards your spine in the correct position, your muscles are literally trained into the ideal position, resulting in a beautiful, flat tummy.

For my pregnancy, I opted for the *Born to Be Beautiful* front plank. It offers most of the benefits of the traditional plank but it is much more comfortable. I did this every morning from the beginning of my pregnancy until I was eight-months pregnant. I resumed it two weeks post pregnancy.

Here's how it's done:

- Gently lower yourself to the floor (in front of a mirror) and get into the all-fours position as seen in the diagram.

- Make sure your back is flat and that your hands and knees are shoulder-width apart.

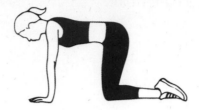

- When you are in the correct position, draw in your tummy, bringing your navel toward your spine. Your back should stay flat at all times; avoid arching it. As you draw in your tummy, breathe out slowly for a count of eight. You should feel a tightening of the tummy area.

- Allow your muscles to relax.

- Repeat twelve times.

Movement 2: The Side Plank

This is a variation of the plank that I recommend you do approximately six weeks post pregnancy. This position is also an isometric exercise but it targets the oblique areas of the abdominals, so it's great for redefining your waist and getting rid of love handles. I do not recommend you do this during pregnancy as it may be too strenuous.

Here's how it's done:

- Begin by lying on your side on the floor in front of a mirror.

- Position your elbow on the floor just under your shoulder.

- Lift up on that elbow and keep your body stiff from head to toe.

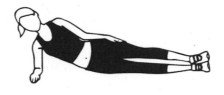

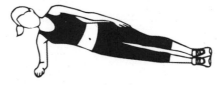

- Hold this position for a count of ten and then lower your hip to the floor.

- Rest and repeat three times.

- Switch sides and repeat the exercise on the other hip.

You can increase the effect of this exercise by lifting the top leg toward the ceiling. Slowly repeat the leg lift ten times and then return to the start position. If you prefer, you can do these exercises on a hand rather than an elbow.

Movement 3: The Side Bend

During pregnancy, this movement was my alternative to the side plank. Here's how it's done:

- Standing in front of a mirror, knees slightly bent and shoulder-width apart, tighten your tummy muscles, drawing your navel towards your spine. As you pull in your tummy, breathe out and slide your right arm towards the floor, keeping your arm close to the right side of your body. Do the stretch slowly, until you feel a slight stretch in the left side of your tummy. Slide back up to the starting position and breathe normally.

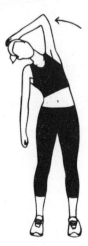

- Switch to the left. Tummy in, breathe out, slide your left arm towards the floor, keeping your arm close to your left side. Do it slowly, until you feel a slight stretch in the right side of your tummy.

- Alternate left and right, ten times per side.

Movement 4: The Scissors

Scissor exercise uses certain leg movements to develop and train various abdominal core muscles. The key for correct use of this type of training is in understanding which type of scissor movements train which muscle groups. We need to target the lower area and the hips.

Here's how it's done:

- Lie on the floor, face-up, with your legs fully extended and your hands under your bottom for extra support.

- To achieve the starting position for the exercise, raise both of your feet six inches from the floor, with your knees slightly bent.

- Once your feet are six inches from the ground, move your legs outward, separating them.

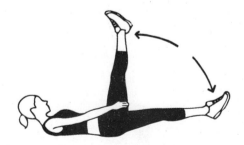

- Briefly hold your legs in this separated position before bringing them back to the starting position. Once together, you can actually cross your feet over each other, alternating which foot is on top with each successive repetition, like scissors midair.

- Do ten scissor movements. Repeat three times.

Movement 5: Pull-ins

This movement can be done anywhere, anytime – even when you're watching TV!
Here's how it's done:

- Sit on a chair. Place both hands on your tummy.

- Inhale and expand your tummy, feeling your hands move out.

- Exhale and contract your abdominal muscles, pulling them in all the way toward your spine. Maintain the contraction for a count of twenty and then do ten quick squeezes.

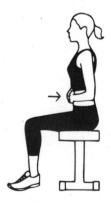

- Repeat three times.

You can apply a less obvious version of this movement to everyday situations. I sometimes did it when I was waiting in a queue at the cinema or in the store, for example. Nobody will notice that you are working your core from within. Simply contract your tummy muscles any time you think of it, no matter where you are.

Movement 6a: The Hula Hoop
This is another really easy to do movement that you can do during and after pregnancy.

Here's how it's done:

- In front of your mirror, knees slightly bent, hands on hips, imagine you have a hula hoop around your waist. Move your hips clockwise in a circular motion, as though spinning it with your waist. Draw in your tummy muscles as you do this.

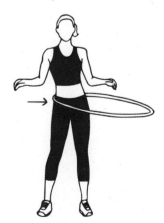

- Repeat ten times clockwise and anticlockwise.

Movement 6b: The Hula Hoop Alternative

An alternative to the hula hoop is to sit upright on a stability ball and roll your hips in a circular motion, ten times clockwise and then ten times anticlockwise, making sure to contract your tummy muscles as you do each movement.

Movement 7: Stability Ball Wall-Squat

This movement is not only great for your core; it is also a great way to tone your legs. I did this every day throughout my pregnancy.

Here's how it's done:

- Place a stability ball between the wall and the curve of your lower back.

- Stand with your feet shoulder-width apart.

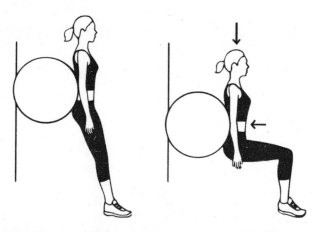

- Bend your knees and lower yourself five to ten inches, shoulders level, hips square. Hold this position for three seconds and then stand up.

- Start with five reps and work up to ten. Rest for thirty seconds and do another set.

Pectoral Strengthening

Your breasts are comprised of fatty adipose tissue and milk glands, not muscle. Therefore you can't firm and tone them per se. However, building and strengthening the pectoral muscles located underneath the breasts is a way to make them appear perky. While many pectoral exercises are done in the gym using equipment, you can do a really good one at home, namely the chest fly. This exercise uses small weights to work the pectoral muscles. You can buy an inexpensive set of three- to five-pound weights if you don't have a set already. Here's how it's done:

- Lie comfortably on the floor with your knees bent.

- Hold a weight in each hand and stretch your arms out to your sides. Gently bring your hands together as if you are hugging a large tree. In peak position, your weights should be almost touching and your palms should be facing each other.

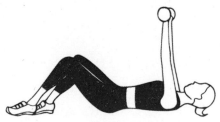

141

- Pause for a few seconds before returning to the starting position. Do three sets of twelve reps.

Dedicate Yourself!

Dedicate yourself to carrying out the *Born to Be Beautiful* movement plan every second day so your body can perform at and look its best. You should begin to notice positive results within a couple of weeks and the results should become more obvious as time goes on.

7

The Born to Be Beautiful Style Guide

Looking and feeling amazing does not mean trying to be something you're not. It means being healthy and happy so you radiate *your* feminine beauty and confidence, enhancing everything you are and all that you have.

When it comes to style, there are three specific things you need to pay attention to: your body shape, your face shape and your colouring. Believe it or not, no matter how good-looking you are, not all clothes, hairstyles and accessories will look good on you, even if they look great on other people.

How well something looks on you and how much it will enhance you is determined by how well what you wear matches your body shape, face shape and colouring. This will become very obvious to you when you implement what I show you in this book. It's like hanging a dress on a hanger. If you try to put a dress on a hanger meant for trousers it will look terrible, but if you put it on a dress-hanger it will look much better.

The clothes you have in your wardrobe may not be the right *match* for you, and how well your clothes match you will determine whether you look average or amazing. Let's make you look amazing!

What Shape Is Your Body?

There are five general body shapes. The natural inclination for many women is to assume they are 'round', which is very unlikely to be the case. Your shape is not determined by how much you weigh. It is determined by a ratio, which we will look at shortly. You might be surprised to find out the shape you actually are.

We will go through each shape below and determine yours. Then we will look at the dos and don'ts for each. As you will see, I have made this very straightforward for you by detailing each one simply and with a graphic. When I ask women to do this at my seminars (see www.donnakennedy.com), they are shocked at how specific changes can make such massive differences to their overall appearances and, consequently, to how they feel!

There Are Five Body Shapes

1. Hourglass
2. Rectangle

3.   Triangle/Pear

4.   Inverted Triangle

5.   Oval

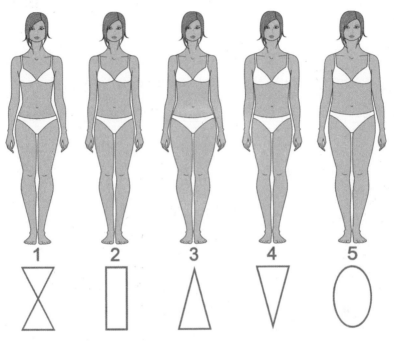

To determine your shape, we simply look at the ratio of your hip line to your bustline, not your overall size. For example, if you have an hourglass figure and you measure your bustline from one side of your chest to the other and your hip line from one hip across to the other, the two measurements will be quite similar, regardless of your current weight. If you are a pear-shape, your hip line will be larger than your bustline, regardless of your weight.

Start by simply measuring your bustline and hip

line. Now match yourself to one of the shapes below, based on the relationship between the two numbers.

Hourglass

- Your full hip line and your full bustline are the same width and your waist is well-defined.

- You most likely have a balanced vertical body shape.

Rectangle

- Your full bustline and full hip line are about the same width and you have little waist definition.

- Your legs and arms will typically be proportionally slender.

- You have a small- to medium-sized bust.

- You most likely have a balanced body or long-legged vertical body shape.

- You may also have a flat bottom.

- You may have had an hourglass figure when you were younger or slimmer.

- You may look shorter and heavier than you really are.

Triangle/Pear

- Your full bustline is proportionally narrower than your full hip line and you have a well-defined waist.

- You typically have narrow shoulders.

- You most likely have a balanced or short-legged vertical body shape.

- Your thighs are typically full.

Inverted Triangle

- You have a proportionally large bust, or you have broad shoulders, or both.

- You have narrow hips with a well-defined waist.

- You most likely have a long-legged vertical body shape with proportionally slim legs.

- You may also have a flat bottom.

Oval

- You have the overall appearance of being round, especially around the waistline.

- Your waistline is undefined.

- You have a large, low stomach.

- You may have 'love handles'.

- You may have a full bottom or a flat bottom.

- Your upper thighs are full.

Dos and Don'ts for Your Body Shape

Now that you have identified your shape, find the relevant style dos and don'ts below. Then simply follow the guidelines, either by giving your wardrobe an overhaul, or bringing your clothes to a seamstress for alterations.

Hourglass

Dos

- Garments that are shapely, especially at the waist

- Soft fabrics

- Garments that emphasise curves without cluttering

- Straight and slightly flared pants and skirts (pencil skirts exaggerate the curve from the hip to the knee)

- Dresses that emphasise the waist

- Tops that are fitted at the waist, wide open at the neckline and have something to divert the eye towards the shoulders, like puffed sleeves

- Simple jewellery

- Jackets with curved lapels to show off curves and three-quarter sleeves to show off elegant wrists and suggest a delicate frame

- Shirts that fasten at the side (do not button all the way to the top)

- Cute shoes with a rounded front, peep toes or bows.

- Make sure that the dress or top fits the bust, as it is easier to take things in at the back.

- Coats with deep 'V's, full skirts and pockets on the hips.

Don'ts

- Stiff fabrics

- Garments that clutter

- Baggy styles

- Skirts with open pleats

- Tapered pants

- Flap side-pockets on trousers
- Big belts
- Batwing sleeves
- Deep V-neck fitted cardigans
- Pointy shoes like stilettos or cowboy boots
- Sleeves that cut in

Rectangle

The aim is to add definition to your shape by visually elongating your body and defining your shoulders (if you are overweight) or defining your waist (if you are slender).

Dos

- Slight shaping of garments
- Classic round-necked jumpers
- Angular jackets that point to your waist
- Shoulder-line emphasis
- Dresses that wrap or flow through the waistline
- Feminine chiffon
- High-waisted dresses, wrap dresses
- Jackets that fasten with tied belts or sashes

- Three-quarter length coats that are belted (like trench coats), tied either at the front or the back, preferably with hip pockets

- Coats that are cut in an Empire line that comes in at the waist

- Straight and semi-fitted jackets and dresses

- Straight or slightly flared flat-fronted pants

- High focal points

- A-line skirts

- Accessories that focus attention on the centre or the top of your body

- Fitted vests with shirts, blouses or T-shirts underneath to carve into the body

- Shapewear that shapes the waist

Don'ts

- Clingy fabrics

- Fitted silhouettes

- Baggy pants

- Big, loose tops

- Narrow skirts

- Cropped tops

- Dropped waists

Triangle/Pear

The aim is to create balance by visually broadening your upper body and slimming your lower body.

Dos

- Horizontal lines on your upper body

- Puff sleeves that broaden the shoulders

- Dresses that are body-hugging on the top, accentuate your tiny waist and then drape outwards, drawing a discreet veil over the width of your thighs (wrap dresses are a great style to try)

- Broad-lapelled jackets and wide-cut necklines

- Cropped jackets

- Jumper worn over shirts, T-shirts or blouses

- Wide-legged or straight pants in a flat-fronted style that hang from the top of your bottom and don't cling to your thighs

- Dark-coloured garments on the lower half of your body to help slim your legs

- Vertical lines on your lower body

- Straight and slightly flared skirts (A-lines are a good choice)

- Shapewear that is like biker pants

Don'ts

- Stiff fabrics

- Shapeless garments

- Side pockets on pants (look out for angled pockets that appear to be straining)

- Full skirts with open pleats

- Pencil skirts

- Tapered pants (like fashionable skinny jeans)

- Jodhpurs (like horse-riding pants)

- Spaghetti-strap tops

- Jackets that cut across the bum

- Cropped trousers (like Capri-style pants)

- Stretch trousers of any kind

- Ankle straps or stilettos

Inverted Triangle

The aim is to create balance by creating the impression of a wider bottom and drawing attention away from the upper body.

Dos

- Horizontal lines for the lower body

- Vertical lines for the upper body
- Draping dresses that curve in all the right places
- Dresses that flow through the waist
- Fluted skirts with flaring hemlines to balance your upper and lower halves
- Draping skirts that gather on the hips
- A-line skirts
- Coats with buttons that sit underneath the bust
- Set-in sleeves
- Side-shaped garments
- Properly fitted bras
- Shapewear that shapes you from bust to the bottom
- Flared pants

Don'ts

- Stiff fabrics
- Garments that emphasise your waist
- Full sleeves
- Big collars
- Tapered pants
- Chunky knit sweaters
- Double-breasted jackets

- Shift dresses

- Polo necks

- High-waisted trousers

- Bolero jackets

- Elaborate necklaces

- Shapeless dresses

- Three-quarter sleeves or sleeves that finish at the bustline

- Cut-away shoulders

- Scooped necklines

- Shoulder pads

Oval

The aim is to visually elongate your body and pull attention toward your head and shoulders. Creating length in your torso will give you a longer, more flattering silhouette.

Dos

- Semi-fitted, boxy and soft silhouettes

- Low necklines

- Tops and blouses worn out

- T-shirts that are rushed in the middle

- Wide V-necks to break up the size of your chest
- Straight duster coats worn against contrasting colours and fabrics, finishing above the knee if you are short
- Vertical design influence, top to bottom
- Properly fitted bras
- Support garments for your torso
- Flat-front, straight and soft pants
- Straight and subtly flared skirts
- Loose-fitting garments
- Dresses that flow through the waistline
- High focal points

Don'ts

- High necklines
- Over-embellishment
- Pleats
- Waist emphasis
- Belts
- Tucked-in tops
- Large lapels
- Full sleeves
- Tight T-shirts

- High-waisted pants

- Pleated waists

- Puffa jackets

- Men's jackets

The Clexy Look

Clexy is a word I use for a classy-sexy combination look – a must for every woman, especially when you are pregnant and possibly struggling to still feel sexy. Allow yourself to stay true to your femininity. Wear clothes with a simple under-bust detail for comfort but stick to your body shape as a general guide. Your body shape does not change when you are pregnant, even with a bump. One of my favourite pregnancy dresses was a red halter-neck dress that had a simple jewelled under-bust sash. The dress was simple and elegant and the halter-neck and jewel details added sexiness.

Face Shapes

Determining the shape of your face is just as important as determining the shape of your body. Face shape determines what haircut suits you best and what accessories (jewellery, glasses and hats) will work for you, all of which will add to your overall look.

Below, we will determine your face shape and then focus on what haircuts are best for your face shape. There is a general rule for accessories and that is simply never repeat the shape of your face in your accessories. For example, if you have a round face, do not wear round jewellery or round glasses. Go for square or long accessories instead.

There Are Six Face Shapes

1. Heart

2. Square

3. Round

4. Diamond

5. Rectangle/Long

6. Oval

What Shape Is Your Face?

To determine the shape of your face, we need to figure out your face ratios. This will be easier to do using a ruler than a tape measure. Write down each of the following five measurements.

1. The width of your forehead at its widest point

2. The width of your cheekbones at their widest

3. Your jawline at its widest point

4. The length of your face, from hairline to chin

5. The width of your face, just under your eyes, starting/stopping where your ears begin

Heart

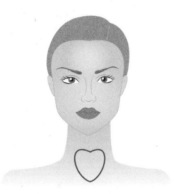

Heart-shaped faces are wider at the forehead and gently narrow down at the jawline. Your chin may be pointy.

Dos

- Short hair, which tends to look great on people with heart-shaped faces. Keep the top layers soft and long. (Note: If you're tall, it's better to go with longer hair, as short hair can create an imbalanced look.)

- You could also choose long hair, if it has long layers that frame your cheekbones.

- A fringe, which will draw attention to your eyes and cheekbones instead of your chin. Side-swept or brow-grazing fringes look great.

Don'ts

- Short, blunt-cut fringes
- Harsh layers

Square

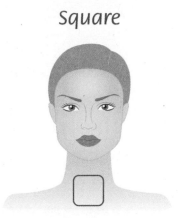

You likely have a square face if you have a strong, angular jawline. The width of your forehead, cheekbones, and jaw are equal, and the ratio of your face's width (ear to ear) to its height (hairline to chin) is 1:1 or 1:1.5. The key is to soften and compliment your strong, angular jawline.

Dos

- Curls, choppy ends or edgy haircuts, which create texture

- Very short, edgy haircuts – unless you are tall
- Long, sleek styles with layers that start at the jawline and continue downwards
- Long bobs
- Side-swept fringes

Don'ts

Single-length bob hairstyles, especially chin-length
Wide, blunt fringes

Round

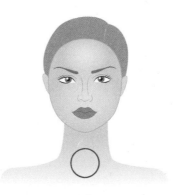

Round faces tend to be soft, with non-angular features and full cheeks. If you have excess weight, you might assume you have a round face, but rely on the ratio guidelines, not your initial assumption. Many round-faced women are thin.

Both round faces and square faces are equal in height and width. The difference is in the angles.

Square faces have strong, angular features, whereas round faces have soft features. You likely have a round face if the following are true.

- Your forehead, cheekbones and jaw are equally wide.
- Your jaw is slightly rounded, rather than angular.
- You have soft features, in general.
- The ratio of your face's width (ear to ear) to its height (hairline to chin) is 1:1.

If you have a round face, the aim is to make it appear longer.

Dos

- Cuts that fall just below the chin, like a long bob
- Soft, graduated layers that make your face appear slimmer and tend to remove bulk and weight from its sides
- Wispy and tapered ends
- Side-swept or long fringes

Don'ts

- Single-length, blunt haircuts such as the classic straight bob
- Short, curly hair

Diamond

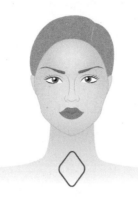

You have a diamond-shaped face if it is widest at the cheekbones, and your jawline and forehead are the same length. The hair styles that will suit you best are the same as those that work for people with square-shaped faces. Again, the aim is to soften and compliment your strong, angular jawline.

Dos

- Curls, choppy ends or edgy cuts
- Very short, edgy cuts – unless you are tall
- Long, sleek styles with layers that start at the jawline and continue downwards
- Long bobs
- Side-swept fringes

Don'ts

- Single-length bobs – especially chin-length
- Wide, blunt fringes

Rectangle

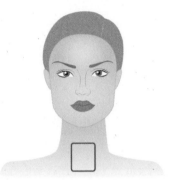

Rectangular faces are longer than they are wide. If the ratio of the width of your face (ear to ear) to the length of your face (hairline to chin) is 1:1.5 or more, then you have a rectangular face. The key is to add width.

Dos

- Fringes that hide the forehead, creating the illusion of a shorter face, including side-swept fringes, grazed fringes and blunt fringes
- Chin-length bobs
- Curls and waves

Don'ts

- Cuts below the collarbone
- cuts that are super short

Oval

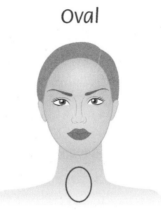

You have an oval-shaped face if the length of your face equals is 1.5 times the width of your face. This is the most versatile shape. You can wear almost any haircut.

Dos

- Most haircuts will work for you but, to get the 'wow' factor, consider your best feature and highlight it with your hair cut. For example, if you have beautiful eyes, a side-swept or blunt fringe can bring attention to them.

Don'ts

- If your hair is thick or curly, avoid a blunt cut.

- If you have curly hair, stay away from short haircuts.

- If you're tall, avoid short hair.

- If you're short, avoid really long hair.

Dress for Your Colouring

Do you have warm, cool or mid-tone colouring? Let's see. Wearing the correct colours to suit your skin tone is essential! You can expand on the colour ranges outlined below by purchasing colour cards, or you could go to a paint store and look at the colour wheels to suit your range.

Warm

You have some red tones in your hair, from rich brown through to auburn or ginger – you may even be strawberry blonde. Your skin tone is a little sallow or freckly, but generally not dark or mid-brown. The colours that suit you are autumnal: those with a golden undertone.

Colours that Suit You Best

- Tomato red

- Light khaki

- Brick red

- Beige
- Tobacco
- Apricot
- Dark coffee
- Olive green
- Green gold
- Deep purple

Colours that Suit You Least

- Dark grey
- Navy
- Silver
- Rose pink
- Hot pink
- Icy blue
- Sky blue

Tip: Your jewellery should be gold or have a warm undertone.

Cool

Your skin is most likely alabaster white or pale with a cool undertone. Your eyes may have dark rims around their irises and may be very dark to mid-brown.

Colours that Suit You Best

- Silver
- Dark grey
- Dove grey
- Blue-red
- Bright emerald
- Bright turquoise
- Navy
- Soft Pink
- Cardinal

Colours that Suit You Least

- Apricot
- Dark coffee
- Olive green
- Light khaki
- Green-gold
- Brick
- Warm reds
- Hot pink

Tip: Your jewellery should be silver or have cool undertones.

Mid-Tone

If you have mid-tone colouring, you veer towards muted bright colours. Too bright and they overwhelm you, too pastel and they drain the colour from your complexion. Without make-up you can appear quite washed-out. When you are looking at your wardrobe, rethink all very cold or very warm colours and the colours that are dirty, like beige or khaki. Your green is a sage, like the fresh, newborn leaf of an olive tree, as opposed to its dying neighbour. If you are choosing purple, avoid that bright, cold tone and go for a dark lavender instead.

Colours that Suit You Best

- Clear red
- Hot pink
- Dark lavender
- Lemon yellow
- Aqua
- Sage
- Medium green
- Periwinkle blue

Colours that Suit You Least

- Rust
- Green-gold
- Salmon
- Warm beige
- Apricot
- Icy blue
- Charcoal
- Black

Tip: Your jewellery should be soft in colour, not bright gold or bright silver.

Making Changes

Now, having identified your body shape, face shape and colouring, you can play around with your haircut and wardrobe. You may need to take your clothes to a seamstress for alteration or maybe invest in some new clothes post pregnancy.

During pregnancy, it can be tricky to get something that doesn't make you look like you're wearing a parachute but, by using the style guide here, you can always look and feel a million dollars. Little tweaks during pregnancy are fine. The same rules generally apply to your shape whether you have a bump at the front or not. Shape is based on ratios, remember, not your pregnancy bump, and your colouring remains fairly constant throughout.

The only real difference during and shortly after pregnancy is that you need to allow extra room for your clothes to stretch over your bump. Buying longer or slightly looser items will make this easy. Obviously, when the bump is gone, you don't need to consider it – just stick to the guide as written here. And look out for my style webinars on my website: www.don-nakennedy.com!

It's Time to Bring Out the Best You!

Don't be afraid to become visible to the world. You are a worthwhile and unique person who deserves to be noted in this world. You deserve to shine and to be seen, to be the best you can be in every way. You were born to be beautiful inside and out.

8
Implement and Maintain

Have you ever read a really great book that taught you lots, and then failed to use any of the information in it? Let's face it: we're all guilty. We've all read that book that we knew could improve our lives. We've all promised ourselves that, when we finished the book, we would return and do the exercises, only to put the book aside and never pick it up again.

I want *Born to Be Beautiful* to be different for you. I want this book to actually make a significant positive impact on your life and your baby's life. I don't want it to just be a good read or a decoration for your book-shelf. This is an opportunity for you to reach your potential, to give yourself and your baby the best. You and your baby deserve it, so it's time now to decide on the outcome you want, to commit to it, and to do what it takes to achieve it. You have the tools to look and feel absolutely amazing, now it's time to use them.

Decide, commit and do.

But ...

Ah yes, the 'but'! We all have at least one, don't we? As human beings, we have been conditioned to put excuses in our way, especially when it comes to change or something that requires effort. Even if taking certain actions will inevitably make our lives better, we just don't seem to allow ourselves the chance to be the best we can be. Instead, we worry about what others might think or what it might mean for us to improve our lives. *Will people comment? What if I fail? Will life change*? And so we find ourselves using our most effective excuses or postponing taking action 'until Monday', which never arrives.

I've Tried Before and It Didn't Work Out, So Why Set Myself Up for Failure Again?

It's understandable that if we tried something and it didn't work out we would hesitate to try it again. But how about looking at failure in a different way? Failure is really just feedback, the world's way of telling us that our strategy wasn't the right one and we need a better one. Think of a fly bashing its head against a closed window, trying to fly out of a room. It does the same thing over and over, getting nowhere in the process. If only it would change the strategy and realise the door is open next to it.

It's all a matter of perspective, being open to new ways of doing things and having a willingness to adjust. Sometimes a shift in thinking and some small actions are all it takes to get an amazing result – but you do need to take action. So don't beat yourself up about past efforts. Think feedback, not failure!

I don't have time

This is a very common excuse for not doing something: 'I am so busy that I just can't find a minute.' We've all used that line at some point. But think about it. Every four years there is a leap year, an extra twenty-four hours handed to us. What did you do with these extra twenty-four hours last leap year? I bet you can't even remember. You see, you do have time, you just need to prioritise better, decide what's most important to you and block off time for it. I'm sure if I told you that in eighteen months I would give you an all-expenses-paid vacation if you found some time to devote to yourself every day, you would manage it quite easily. The world will not fall apart because you take time out. Prioritise yourself and your baby.

I'm Not Confident Like Other People

We can compare ourselves to women who do something so much easier and quicker than we do, but the fact is that confidence is not a thing that some people have and some people don't. It is situation-dependent. For example, I am confident in my ability to write but I am not confident in my ability to have a conversation in Chinese. You see, we only become confident when we do something more than once and it works out the way we want. Those people you see who are confident public speakers, confident drivers and super socialites, they learned it and practiced it until it became natural, which means you can become confident in whatever you want to be confident in – if you do it enough times. If looking and feeling amazing is what you want, just do what is written in this book and keep doing it until you get the result you want. And you will get it! For additional support look out for my confidence webinars on my website: www.donnakennedy.com.

The Recumbent Bike

Think of working toward your goal as hopping on a recumbent bike, like the ones used in spin classes. Initially, when you get on, it may be tough to get the wheels spinning. You have to expend a little energy and work against some resistance, whether physical or emotional. But once you push past those first few tough seconds and gather momentum, it's easy, and soon your legs are spinning away using far less energy than it took to get started. Those women you envy, who seem to have that indescribable ease and consistency in pregnancy and motherhood, actually just got started and created momentum. They started the process and kept going until it became easy. Sure, getting started can be tough, or at least different. But once you push past the effort required at the beginning, even the smallest successes can build upon one another, creating an eventual tidal wave of momentum pushing you onward and upward towards your desired outcome.

As the American suffragette Frances Willard said, 'The world is wide, and I will not waste my life in friction when it could be turned into momentum.' Intuitively, we know momentum is needed to achieve a goal. It's what helps us avoid distractions and bounce back from setbacks. It's what sees us through from our initial, inspired excitement to the routine of daily actions needed to keep us on course through to the endpoint at which our goal is realised. If we can keep moving on our little projects every day, stoking that positive fire regularly to keep the flames high, so to speak, it's infinitely easier to stay focused, make great strides and blast through any obstacles that come up.

Cultivating Momentum

For most of us, momentum doesn't come automatically but it can be cultivated. Here are some ways that you can create momentum:

1. **State your goal positively**. Rather than describe your desired outcome as a problem or something to get rid of ('I don't want to be overweight and unhealthy' or 'I don't want to feel bad about myself'), frame it as a positive statement that calls to you ('I want to be fit and healthy' or 'I want to feel confident and self-assured'). An outcome stated in the positive form gets your brain excited to take the specific actions needed to achieve it.

2. **Focus on what you can do, not on what you can't do**. Sustaining momentum is all about keeping your eye on the goal and focusing on what *is* possible. You'll encounter obstacles, but don't go looking for them. Keep your focus on what you *can* do and what *is* possible. Take the next step, no matter how small, that will move you forward. As Henry Ford said, 'Obstacles are those frightful things you see when you take your eyes off your goal.'

3. **Picture your perfect result**. Remember, if you want something, visualise it. If you can't

already see it in your mind's eye, how can you really and truly go after what you want? To make it easier to create a perfect mental picture of you attaining your goals, you could create a collage using visual cues such as pictures or pictures of words that trigger an emotional response. It will inspire you and keep you on track. Put that creative collage up somewhere where you'll see it every day, maybe on your fridge or on your phone as a screensaver. Look at the visual cues and really absorb them. Take mere seconds out of your day, in the morning before you get out of bed, or before you go to sleep at night, close your eyes, and really picture yourself achieving what you want. Bring up the lovely emotions that you'll feel when you finally achieve your goal and think about how you'll reward yourself afterwards.

4. **Avoid trying to do everything at once**. To maintain momentum, it's important to break your main goal into small, manageable steps (as we did in Chapter 2), and then take action, one step at a time, every single day. You will avoid overwhelming yourself with your main goal by deconstructing it into digestible parts.

5. **Carve out a consistent block of time to work on yourself**. This is especially important

if you're juggling work or other commitments. Make sure you have regular time to devote to yourself and your goal every day. Although that may be challenging, it's doable. Consistent action is paramount for many reasons: it keeps your head clear and focused, it rewards you with a constant feeling of progress and, most importantly, it keeps the ball moving forward. Don't wait for this free time to magically open up. It won't. Rather, proactively carve out and prioritise a block of time in your daily schedule, make it public, and honour the commitment the same way you would an appointment with your health-care provider.

6. **Understand what it takes to keep you motivated.** There's intrinsic and extrinsic motivation. For example, achievement motivates some people, while social connection motivates others. Positive motivation works for many (rewards), while negative motivation is the ticket for others (avoidance). Think about what it takes to keep you motivated and then leverage that understanding about what makes you tick.

7. **Surround yourself with as many positive people as you can**. Surround yourself with

people who are positive and successful at setting and achieving goals. Being around supportive people is inspiring and helps you raise the bar for yourself. Their goals don't have to be the same as yours but being around them will give you a regular reminder that you can achieve your goal and will help you to focus on your achievements rather than your setbacks.

8. **Think 'active'**. Pursue positive momentum by continually setting short-term, daily goals. Being driven and consistent every single day takes work – life happens – but to keep that powerful momentum from waning, you have to practise discipline. So, once in a while, especially on those inevitable tough days, you may have to suck it up and *just do it*. Seeing your baby smiling at you can motivate you. It will spur you on.

9. **Live without excuses**. Bottom line: there are *always* excuses. There will always be too little time, too many commitments and too many people pulling you in too many directions. Get real with yourself. If you let these excuses get in your way, you'll never even get started and you'll definitely never build momentum. The people who drop excuses from their lives have the most momentum and, inevitably, the most

success. Focus on the fact that you will look and feel amazing as a result of your actions.

10. **Embrace it**. Once you really get some momentum going, don't be afraid of it. Instead, feel good about it and embrace it. As the author Seth Godin said:

> 'Many of us fear too much momentum. We look at a project launch or a job or another new commitment as something that might get out of control. It's one thing to be a folk singer playing to a hundred people a night in a coffeehouse, but what if the momentum builds and you become a star? A rock star? With an entourage and appearances and higher than high expectations for your next work? … Deep down, this potential for an overwhelming response alerts the lizard brain and we hold back.'

11. **Don't hold back**. When it comes to goal execution, the key is to get moving and keep moving. Give yourself the opportunity to be the best you can be.

12. **Regularly review your overall progress and reorient toward your goal**. If you were taking a trip across the country and took a wrong turn, you wouldn't just keep going,

wandering aimlessly. You'd stop, reorient yourself and get back on track. Do the same for your goal. Map out your course, keeping track of where you are and making course adjustments as necessary. Refer often to your goal template from Chapter 2.

13. **Celebrate your successes, big or small**. You can build on success more easily than on setbacks. Take note of every step forward, no matter how small, and celebrate every milestone. Being aware of and acknowledging your progress sustains your efforts.

Revisiting Your Goals

Rewrite your goals using the template below, and then put the template where you will see it often.

12-Month Goal

_____

_____

_____

_____

_____

_____

_____

_____

_____

_____

_____

_____

6-Month Goal

_____

_____

_____

_____

_____

_____

_____

_____

_____

_____

3-Month Goal

_____

_____

_____

_____

_____

_____

_____

_____

_____

_____

1-Month Goal

_____

_____

_____

_____

_____

_____

_____

_____

_____

_____

_____

_____

1-Week Goal

_____

_____

_____

_____

_____

_____

_____

_____

_____

_____

Today's Goal

_____

_____

_____

_____

_____

_____

_____

_____

_____

_____

_____

Ride the Wave of Momentum

Once you've started and you've gained a little momentum, you can let it work *for* you. Of course, you still have to hold up your end of the bargain by being consistent. Be a turtle. Slow and steady wins the race. Clichéd as it is, that old adage holds true when it comes to momentum. We all know the story from when we were kids. Whereas the careless hare stops and starts over and over again, constantly losing momentum and making it harder each time to start up again, the turtle steadily keeps on keeping on, slowly and at a healthy pace but gaining and maintaining momentum … and we all know how that race ends. Here are some tips for maintaining momentum.

1. **Monitor your progress on a continuous basis**. It's really important that you pay attention to your little milestones as you work your way towards your bigger goal. It's common to get excited at the beginning of any lifestyle change, only to let things slip after a few weeks. Focus on implementing and monitoring your daily actions, ticking the boxes, so to speak. This will keep you on track and give you a sense of accomplishment every day, spurring you on. You don't need to put pressure on yourself to do everything perfectly and brilliantly. Just start and take little steps.

2. **Understand obstacles**. As you implement the *Born to Be Beautiful* plan, you will inevitably meet obstacles. Life happens. Don't be naive and think that you will have no hiccups for the next eighteen months. An off day, bad news, a confrontation, a teething baby, a sleepless night – many things can ruffle our feathers and potentially cause momentum to wane. Understand that you may at some point get blown off course and, if you do, you should simply stop, reorient and refocus. Adjust and take the first step again. The important step is always the first one.

3. **Think long-term**. The *Born to Be Beautiful* plan is about maintaining results long-term. You need to create a lifestyle habit, not try to do everything all at once in fifth gear. The small steps are often the most powerful. Every time you take a small step toward your goal, your brain gets a clear message that the actions you are taking are important and it creates a habit – it sets up an automatic response for positive results. In fact, the *Born to Be Beautiful* plan extends well beyond pregnancy. It can become an enjoyable and healthy way of life for you and your baby for as long as you like.

So, which kind of person do you want to be: the one who gets stuck in a rut fighting inaction, trying to impress and ultimately ending up in a static state or the proactive one who implements information steadily and consistently to get results? Now that you have the tools to make yourself look and feel amazing, choose the latter, *start today*, build momentum and enjoy the results! I will be rooting for you one hundred percent and happy in the knowledge that you now know and appreciate that you and your baby truly were *Born to Be Beautiful*!

Appendix
Born to Be Beautiful
Recipes

The following snacks are some of the ones I ate during my pregnancy. They can be put together very easily and are very nutritious. Make sure to keep some in your fridge, freezer or cupboard at all times so you always have something healthy to fill you, in case you get the munchies.

Butter Bean Salad with Sun-Dried Tomatoes, Olives and Basil Vinaigrette

Ingredients

- 2 cans (425 grams each) of butter beans or any type of white bean
- 1/2 cup sun-dried tomatoes in oil
- 1/2 cup pitted Kalamata olives
- 1/3 cup basil vinaigrette
- 2 to 3 tbsp chopped fresh basil (optional)

Instructions

- To make the basil vinaigrette, combine at room temperature three parts of your favourite low-sugar vinaigrette dressing and one part basil puree.
- Put the basil in the food processor, turn it on and pour the dressing through the feed tube.
- Process until the basil is in very small pieces and completely integrated into the dressing. You should still be able to see some basil pieces but they will be very small.

- To make the salad, drain the beans into a colander placed in the sink, rinse them well with cold water (until no more foam appears) and then let them drain for a minute or two. Blot them dry with paper towels and put them in a medium-sized salad bowl.

- Add about half the basil vinaigrette to the beans and allow to marinate.

- Drain the sun-dried tomatoes to remove the oil and then coarsely chop them.

- Cut the Kalamata olives in half.

- Mix together the marinated beans, sun-dried tomatoes and Kalamata olives.

- Add the rest of the dressing, or as much as you need to moisten the ingredients, then gently mix in the additional chopped basil.

- This salad can be served right away or marinated in the fridge for a few hours. It will keep in the fridge for several days, but you might want to mix in a little extra dressing to refresh the flavours.

Spanish Omelette

This is one of my favourite things to eat. It's really filling and a great way to get a healthy mix of protein and carbs. It is lovely hot or cold with salad.

Ingredients

- 4 eggs (take the yolk out of two of them for a healthier mixture)
- 2 tsp olive oil
- 1 small onion, chopped
- 1 medium potato, cooked, halved and thinly sliced
- Salt and pepper to taste
- Chilli sauce to taste

Instructions

- Break the eggs into a medium-sized bowl or measuring jug. Beat until well combined. Add the salt, pepper and chilli sauce. Mix.
- Heat the frying pan to medium. Add the oil and onion, cook until almost golden and then add the potato. Cook for three minutes.
- Make sure the potato and onion are spread evenly over the pan and then gently pour the

omelette mix into the pan and leave it for five or ten minutes. Keep checking that the bottom doesn't burn.

- Set the grill to medium. When the omelette is half-cooked (when you wiggle the pan and not too much egg slides on the top), place the pan under the grill.

- Check often until the top is golden brown. It should only be a couple of minutes.

- Remove the omelette from the grill and cut it into portions of the desired size.

Quinoa-Stuffed Peppers

This protein-rich dish freezes well for future meals.

Ingredients

- 1 cup finely chopped onion
- 2 tbsp olive oil
- ½ cup finely chopped celery
- 1 tbsp ground cumin
- 2 tsp garlic, minced
- 280 grams frozen, chopped spinach, thawed and squeezed dry
- 850 grams canned diced tomatoes, drained, liquid reserved
- 425 grams canned black beans, rinsed and drained
- ¾ cup quinoa
- 1 ½ cups grated carrots
- 4 large, red bell peppers, halved lengthwise, ribs removed
- 4 tbsp low-fat shredded cheese

Instructions

- Heat the oil in a saucepan over medium heat.

Add the onion and celery and cook for five minutes or until soft. Add the cumin and garlic and sauté for one minute. Stir in the spinach and tomatoes. Cook for five minutes or until most of the liquid has evaporated.

- Stir in the black beans, quinoa, carrots and two cups of water. Cover and bring to a boil. Reduce the heat to medium-low, and simmer for twenty minutes or until the quinoa is tender. Season with salt and pepper, if desired.

- Preheat the oven to 180 degrees. Pour the liquid from the tomatoes into the bottom of the baking dish.

- Fill each bell pepper with about three quarters of a cup of quinoa mixture and then place them all in the baking dish. Cover them with foil and bake them for one hour.

- Uncover and sprinkle each pepper with one tablespoon of low-fat cheese. Bake for fifteen minutes more, or until the tops are browned.

- Let the peppers stand for five minutes. Transfer them to serving plates and drizzle each with pan juices before serving.

Chickpea Pita Bread Pockets

Chickpea pita bread pockets, which are best made of ahead of time, are really refreshing, filling and easy to eat. No excuses!

Ingredients

- 1/4 cup extra-virgin olive oil
- 1 tsp lemon zest
- 2 tbsp lemon juice
- 2 tbsp chopped flat-leaf parsley
- 1 clove garlic, minced
- 1t sp ground cumin
- 1/2 tsp kosher salt
- 1/4 tsp smoked paprika
- 3 cups cooked and drained chickpeas or 30 ounces canned chickpeas
- 1 cup yogurt (preferably Greek-style)
- 2 tbsp chopped mint
- 4 pita bread rounds, lightly toasted or warmed, if desired
- 8 cups chard, spinach or lettuce cut into quarter-inch ribbons

- 3 to 4 tomatoes, sliced
- ½ a red onion, thinly sliced
- Parsley and mint leaves for garnish (optional)

Instructions

- In a bowl, whisk together olive oil, lemon zest, lemon juice, parsley, garlic, cumin, salt and paprika.

- Add the chickpeas and stir to combine. The longer the chickpeas marinate, the better they taste, so if you have time, cover and refrigerate them for at least an hour and up to a couple of days.

- In a separate bowl, combine the yogurt and mint. Again, this is better if it sits for a while, so cover and refrigerate it if you're not using it immediately.

- Cut the pita breads in half. Line each half with chard or other greens and fill them all with tomatoes, chickpeas and onions.

- Garnish with parsley and mint, if desired. Serve with mint yogurt spooned on top.

Hummus and Vegetable Pita Pocket

Ingredients

- 1 whole-wheat pita pocket
- 1/2 cup hummus
- 1/8 cup diced cucumber
- 1/8 cup diced tomato
- 1/8 cup chopped bell pepper
- 1/8 cup shoestring carrots
- 1 slice red onion
- Alfalfa sprouts
- Lettuce

Instructions

- Spread the hummus inside the pita pocket.
- Add assorted veggies.
- Add the lettuce last.
- Enjoy!

Soup

There are many different kinds of soup but my favourite is broccoli. When I was pregnant, I often made a large pot of broccoli soup and stored tubs of it in the freezer. If I felt hungry, it was as easy as heating up some of the soup I had stored. Feel free to eat as much soup as you like and try various flavours. Your stomach digests it very easily.

Ingredients

- 700 grams fresh broccoli
- 1 large onion, chopped
- 1 carrot, chopped
- Salt and freshly ground black pepper
- 4 cups vegetable stock

Instructions

- Sauté the chopped onion in olive oil until it is translucent.
- Add the broccoli, carrot, salt and pepper and cook for about three minutes.
- Add the stock and bring to boil.
- Simmer uncovered until the broccoli is tender, about fifteen minutes.

- With an immersion blender, puree the soup and the pour back into the pot. Add salt and pepper to taste and then put the lid back on the pot.

- Serve hot with homemade croutons or whole-meal bread.

- Voila, simple as that!

Vegetable Samosas

Ingredients

- 2 raw medium-sized potatoes, peeled and diced
- 1 raw small carrot, finely chopped
- 1 small onion, finely chopped
- 50 grams peas, boiled
- ½ tsp ground cumin
- ½ tsp coriander, dried
- ¼ tsp chilli powder
- ¼ tsp turmeric
- 1 tsp garlic, pureed
- 1 tbsp fresh coriander or mint, chopped
- A small pinch of salt
- ¼ tsp black pepper
- 5 sheets filo pastry

Instructions

- Cook the potatoes and carrot in boiling water until they are tender – about ten minutes. Drain and partially mash them.

- Mist a non-stick frying pan with cooking spray.

Add the onion and cook until softened – about two minutes.

- Stir the onion, peas, cumin, ground coriander, chilli powder, turmeric, garlic puree and fresh coriander or mint into the potatoes and carrots. Season to taste. Cool completely.

- Preheat the oven to 180 degrees. Mist your baking sheets with cooking oil.

- Cut the filo pastry sheets into strips measuring approximately thirty centimetres by ten centimetres.

- Place a tablespoon of mixture at one end of a pastry strip. Fold it over and over to make a triangle. Repeat this to make twenty samosas.

- Mist the samosas with cooking spray, place them onto baking sheets and bake them for twenty-five to thirty minutes, until golden.

Thai Fried Rice with Toasted Cashews

Ingredients

- 50 grams of dried Thai jasmine rice
- Calorie-controlled cooking spray
- 1 cm piece fresh root ginger, cut into thin strips
- 6 cashew nuts
- 1 tsp soy sauce
- 2 spring onions, sliced diagonally
- 1 clove garlic, chopped
- 1 stalk lemongrass, peeled and chopped finely
- ½ red chilli, de-seeded and chopped
- 2 fresh coriander sprigs, leaves only

For the dressing

- 1 tbsp soy sauce
- 1 tsp lime juice

Instructions

- Put the rice in a lidded pan and pour in enough cold water to cover by one centimetre. Bring to the boil and then reduce the heat to its lowest setting. Cover and simmer for about ten minutes until the rice is tender and the water is absorbed. Remove from the heat. Leave to stand for five minutes, still covered. Spread the rice out on a baking tray. Leave to cool.

- Heat a non-stick wok or frying pan and spray with the cooking spray. Add the ginger and stir-fry for three minutes, until crisp and golden. Remove from the pan and set aside.

- Put the cashew nuts in the pan, spray them with cooking spray and toast them at medium-low heat for two minutes, turning them frequently. Add the soy sauce and turn the nuts until they are coated. Cook them for another minute until golden then remove from the pan and set aside.

- Wipe the pan, spray it with the cooking spray and then stir-fry the white parts of the spring onions, garlic, lemongrass and chilli for a minute. Add the cold rice, turn it to break up any lumps and combine it with the other ingredients.

- Mix together soy sauce, lime juice and sugar. Pour into the pan, stir and heat through. Stir the green part of the spring onion into the rice. Serve topped with the coriander, cashew nuts and crisp ginger.

Yummy Fajitas

Ingredients

- 4 whole-wheat tortillas
- 2 tsp olive oil
- 2 cloves garlic, minced
- 2 green bell peppers, sliced
- 2 yellow bell peppers, sliced
- 1 onion, sliced
- 1 cup mushrooms, sliced
- 3 green onions chopped
- Lemon pepper to taste

Instructions:

- In a large frying pan over a medium heat, sauté the olive oil and garlic for two minutes.
- Stir in the green and yellow bell peppers and sauté them for two minutes.
- Stir in the onions and, after two minutes, add the mushrooms and green onions.
- Season the vegetables with lemon pepper and stir well.

- Cover the frying pan and cook until all of the vegetables are tender.

- Warm the tortilla wraps, fill and enjoy!

Banana Omelette

I know it sounds gross but try it, you'll like it!

Ingredients

- 2 tsp olive oil
- 2 eggs
- 1 banana

Instructions

- Blend the eggs and banana until smooth.
- Heat the olive oil in a frying pan, pour the mixture in and cook until golden.
- Serve hot.

Supercharged
Born to Be Beautiful Beauty Smoothie

Ingredients

- 1 cup frozen mixed berries
- 2 tbsp natural yoghurt
- ½ banana
- 1 tbsp chia seed
- ½ tsp wheatgrass powder
- ½ tsp spirulina powder
- 250 ml orange juice

Instructions

- Blend ingredients and serve cold.

- You can make smoothie ice pops by pouring some mixture into ice-pop moulds and freezing them.

- As an alternative to berry mix, you could use a mango and pineapple mixture with a dash of lime. It's equally divine!